THE BIOMEDICAL QUALITY AUDITOR HANDBOOK

Also available from ASQ Quality Press:

Quality Audit Handbook, Second Edition
ASQ Quality Audit Division

Quality Audits for Improved Performance, Third Edition
Dennis R. Arter

How to Audit the Process-Based QMS
Dennis R. Arter, Charles A. Cianfrani, and John E. (Jack) West

The Internal Auditing Pocket Guide
J. P. Russell

After the Quality Audit: Closing the Loop on the Audit Process, Second Edition
J. P. Russell and Terry Regel

Internal Quality Auditing
Denis Pronovost

The Quality Auditor's HACCP Handbook
ASQ Food, Drug, and Cosmetic Division

The ISO 9000 Auditor's Companion and *The Audit Kit*
Kent A. Keeney

To request a complimentary catalog of ASQ Quality Press publications, call (800) 248-1946, or visit our Web site at http://qualitypress.asq.org.

THE BIOMEDICAL QUALITY AUDITOR HANDBOOK

Biomedical Division of the
American Society for Quality

Bruce Haggar, Editor

ASQ Quality Press
Milwaukee, Wisconsin

American Society for Quality, Quality Press, Milwaukee 53203

© 2003 by ASQ

All rights reserved. Published 2003

Printed in the United States of America

12 11   5 4

Library of Congress Cataloging-in-Publication Data

The biomedical quality auditor handbook / Bruce Haggar, editor.
     p. cm.
   Includes bibliographical references and index.
   ISBN 0-87389-576-2 (hardcover : alk. paper)
     1. Medical instruments and apparatus—Quality control—Handbooks,
manuals, etc. I. Haggar, Bruce, 1952–

   R856.6.B55 2003
   681'.761'0685—dc21   2003006529

ISBN 0-87389-576-2

Publisher: William A. Tony
Acquisitions Editor: Annemieke Koudstaal
Project Editor: Paul O'Mara
Production Administrator: Gretchen Trautman
Special Marketing Representative: Robin Barry

ASQ Mission: The American Society for Quality advances individual, organizational, and community excellence worldwide through learning, quality improvement, and knowledge exchange.

Attention Bookstores, Wholesalers, Schools and Corporations: ASQ Quality Press books, videotapes, audiotapes, and software are available at quantity discounts with bulk purchases for business, educational, or instructional use. For information, please contact ASQ Quality Press at 800-248-1946, or write to ASQ Quality Press, P.O. Box 3005, Milwaukee, WI 53201-3005.

To place orders or to request a free copy of the ASQ Quality Press Publications Catalog, including ASQ membership information, call 800-248-1946. Visit our Web site at www.asq.org or http://qualitypress.asq.org .

 Printed on acid-free paper

American Society for Quality

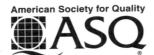

Quality Press
600 N. Plankinton Avenue
Milwaukee, Wisconsin 53203
Call toll free 800-248-1946
Fax 414-272-1734
www.asq.org
http://qualitypress.asq.org
http://standardsgroup.asq.org
E-mail: authors@asq.org

Table of Contents

Preface

The *Biomedical Quality Auditor Handbook* was written to serve as a source of information and knowledge for application of quality auditor principles to the biomedical industry. The Biomedical Division has long believed that in order for auditors and other biomedical professionals to be effective in their jobs, the information they need to be aware of is very extensive. Interpretations of that information vary widely from industry to industry, and specific auditing skills and knowledge may be more important in the medical industry because of its highly regulated nature. This book provides descriptions of a wide range of subjects that have specific interpretations unique to the biomedical industry. This book, which provides industry-specific interpretation, can be used in conjunction with the *Quality Audit Handbook* published by the Quality Audit Division, which provides information on basic auditor skills.

The information in this book is based on a body of knowledge established by the Biomedical Division that was current at the time the book was written. However, that body of knowledge is constantly being changed because it contains references to standards and guidance documents that are constantly evolving. The Biomedical Division intends to publish updates to the body of knowledge as required. Those updates will be published on the Biomedical Division Web site and on the ASQ Web site for reference.

This book does not address ISO 9001:2000 in detail due to the large amount of information published on the subject and available through ASQ.

It is important to note that much information that readers may consider important knowledge in the biomedical field may not be dealt with in this book. This book is intended to support the body of knowledge and not provide additional information. The body of knowledge was prepared based on surveys and careful evaluation.

The Biomedical Division believes that this publication will be a valuable reference to those biomedical professionals. The Division's primary mission is education, both of our members and those associated with the industry. We hope this text helps to fulfill that mission.

Bruce Haggar

Notes to the Reader

Each topic in the book, and in many cases a part of a topic, was written by an individual author. The authors were asked to follow current guidance and the body of knowledge while writing their sections. In many cases the authors were well aware of upcoming changes to the documents contained in the body of knowledge and generally followed the existing guidance, not the expected guidance.

The topics in this book are described in summary fashion. There is just too much information for each topic to be dealt with in a complete fashion in a single text. Even the documents listed as references in the bibliography are only that and not the complete set of information available. The authors used their discretion in writing their sections.

It is the reader's obligation to ensure that he or she is aware of and reads the reference material and other topic material in order to have a complete background in any one topic. We believe that with this text and with the reference materials, readers can have a well-rounded background in the biomedical field.

Acknowledgments

A number of individuals helped write this book, and the Biomedical Division and I appreciate that effort. The participants are division members who are widely regarded as industry experts in specific areas. We thank all of them for their participation.

Contributing authors include:

Elizabeth Blackwood, Johnson and Johnson, who contributed to sections on the Quality System Regulation and other 21 Code of Federal Regulations.

David Dunn, Celera Diagnostics, who contributed to the sections on in-vitro diagnostics.

Sue Jacobs, QMS Consulting, Inc., who contributed to the Quality System Regulation, other 21 CFR regulations, and the quality system inspection technique.

Don Johnson, Cooltouch, Inc., who contributed to the sections on sterilization and biocompatibility.

Dan Olivier, Certified Software Solutions, Inc., who contributed to the sections on risk management and software development.

Susan Reilly, Reilly and Associates, who contributed to the sections on the Quality System Regulation and international auditing guidelines.

Mark Roberts, Roberts Consulting and Engineering, who contributed to the sections on international quality system guidance and international quality system standards.

Steve Thompson, Curagen Corporation, who contributed to the sections on laboratory testing.

Jim Wood, Reed Smith Crosby Heafy, who contributed to the section on base U.S. law.

Bruce Haggar, Med Q Systems, Inc., who contributed to the sections on the Quality System Regulation, U.S. compliance programs, and controlled environments and utility systems.

The Biomedical Division would also like to acknowledge Keith Rohrbach, who headed the division's activities to develop the body of knowledge and biomedical quality auditor certification.

Part I

U.S. Base Law and Regulations

Chapter 1

Base U.S. Law

FDA REGULATION OF MEDICAL DEVICES

The Federal Food, Drug, and Cosmetic Act (FDCA) allows for extensive regulation of medical devices. The FDCA currently governs the entire life span of a device, from premarket certification, through the manufacturing process, subsequent release to the market, and use by the consumer. However, Congress's original Food and Drugs Act did not govern medical devices.

The Federal Food and Drugs Act, promulgated in 1906, regulated only drugs and not medical devices. After repealing the act in 1938, Congress recast it as the FDCA, adding specific provisions for enforcement actions concerning devices. However, the actions were limited to policing post-market activity through prohibition of adulteration and misbranding. The 1938 act did not provide for premarket review or post-market surveillance of devices. When Congress amended the act in 1962, it still did not include provisions for those regulatory activities.

With the passage of the Medical Device Amendments of 1976 (MDA), Congress expanded the Food and Drug Administration's (FDA) authority to regulate devices. One significant change was a broadened definition of "device." The term included "implements, machines, implants, in vitro reagents, and other similar or related articles."[1] Additionally, the MDA increased the conditions that qualified a device for regulation under the FDCA. Inclusion in the National Formulary or the U. S. Pharmacopeia (USP), or any supplement documents, became qualifying criteria. The definition of "device" was also fine-tuned by adding limitations. To be regulated by the MDA, a device must neither: 1) "achieve any of its principal intended purposes through chemical action within or on the body of humans or animals," or 2) be "dependent upon being metabolized for the achievement of any of its principal intended purposes."[2]

The MDA gave the FDA authority to inspect devices. This authority included new requirements that device manufacturers or importers maintain records and provide reports to assure that devices were safe and effective. Additionally, FDA representatives could physically inspect the materials, facilities, equipment, and vehicles used for manufacturing or transporting devices.[3]

The MDA also granted the FDA the power to control the commercial release of medical devices. The amendments created a three-tiered scheme for premarket regulation and post-market review. For this purpose, devices were divided into three classes, based upon their perceived safety risk. Class I devices, those deemed to pose the least risk of harm, were to be the least regulated, while Class III would be the most heavily regulated.

The MDA provided two procedures by which devices could receive approval for release. They were 510(k) premarket notifications and premarket approval applications (PMAs). The FDA was also granted the authority to impose performance standards and to ban devices entirely.

More than 10 years later, Congress passed the Safety Medical Devices Act of 1990 (SMDA) to enhance the FDA's regulation of devices. This new legislation followed in the wake of criticism by congressional investigators and others of the limits of the earlier act. The SMDA imposed more stringent premarket and post-market requirements, as well as new mechanisms for enforcement. Now the FDA must issue an order of approval before a manufacturer can market a device pursuant to a 510(k) notification. The SMDA also added the authority for the FDA to set performance standards. Further, it included a provision allowing post-market surveillance of Class II or III devices that may pose serious health risks, are life supporting or sustaining, or are meant to be implanted in humans for more than one year. Additionally, the FDCA added the civil penalties to the FDA's enforcement options.

The device statutes of the FDCA had two further revisions in the 1990s. The Medical Device Amendments of 1992 did not include major changes to existing device law. However, the FDA Modernization Act of 1997 is notable for the progressiveness of two of its statutes. Both provide greater access to state-of-the-art device technology. The first provision permits device manufacturers and distributors to disseminate information to medical practitioners and insurers concerning new uses for devices already in commercial distribution. Permissible information is limited to peer-reviewed articles or reference publications based on clinical investigation.[4] The companion statute allows shipment of investigational devices in emergency situations or to combat serious conditions.[5] The law further enables patients being treated by licensed physicians to request and receive these devices directly from the manufacturer or distributor. Both of these provisions reflect a major shift for the FDCA. Since its inception, the amendments to the FDCA imposed tighter restrictions on distribution of devices in the interest of safety. Here, the countervailing interest of allowing greater access to medical advances is balanced against the FDCA's primary safety concerns.

SUMMARY OF MEDICAL DEVICE MISBRANDING REGULATIONS

Prohibitions against misbranding and adulteration are two longstanding consumer safeguards provided by the FDCA. Both were included in the original Pure Food and Drug Act of 1906.[6] *Misbranding regulations* protect against the sale of unregistered and exceptionally risky devices, as well as against false or insufficient statements appearing in product packaging or advertisements. *Adulteration laws* are intended to ensure that a device conforms to its original certification, and continues to meet that standard throughout its life.

For purposes of this section, it is important to note that Section 520 of the FDCA creates a category for devices that are restricted. These are devices that are limited by regulation to sole distribution or use by authorization of a licensed practitioner or by other conditions imposed by the FDA.

Through misbranding statutes, device manufacturers are prohibited from making misrepresentations about the product and are required to disclose specific types of information to potential users, as well as to the FDA. The laws forbid the inclusion of misstatements in product labeling and advertisements. Additionally, these materials must identify the product's origin, uniform product descriptions, and instructions for safe use. Finally, misbranding statutes may require producers and distributors of high-risk devices to issue notifications of unreasonable risks or to conduct post-market surveillance.

Misbranding provisions concerning product origin protect the public from purchasing devices that have not been properly registered. A product may be characterized as misbranded if it is disseminated without the product origin information that has been mandated by the FDA, or if it originates from a producer that has failed to register either its facilities or a device with the agency.[7] The FDA requires that product packaging identify the name and place of business of device manufacturers, packers, and/or distributors.[8] In addition, a properly branded device is one for which the following procedures have been followed: 1) it was manufactured, prepared, propagated, compounded, and/or processed in a facility registered in compliance with FDCA regulations;[9] 2) it was included on the facility's registered list of devices for commercial distribution;[10] and 3) before the device was introduced into interstate commerce, the producer notified the FDA of the device's classification, as well as the producer's efforts to comply with performance standards and premarket approval requirements.[11]

In contrast to the detailed product origin requirements, the misbranding restrictions also forbid inclusion of false or misleading information in device labeling or advertisements.[12] A device is misbranded if it is dangerous when used in the manner, frequency, or duration suggested, prescribed, or recommended in its labeling.[13] If the device is a restricted one, the prohibition against false or misleading statements extends to advertisements.[14]

The regulations also include a duty to submit product labeling for review by the secretary of health and human services. The amount of material to be submitted depends on whether the device is restricted or is subject to a performance standard or premarket approval requirements. Producers and distributors of devices that do not fall into those categories are simply obliged to provide the secretary with the label and package insert, as well as a representative sampling of any other labeling.[15] All other producers and distributors have the greater obligation of providing a copy of all device labeling.[16] Those producing and distributing restricted devices must submit a representative sample of product advertisements and, upon good cause, the Secretary may request that they provide a copy of all product advertisements.[17]

In addition to outlawing false statements, the FDA requires the inclusion of statements that create greater uniformity in labeling. For example, device packaging must accurately state the weight, measure, or numerical count of its contents.[18] It must also include symbols from the FDA's uniform system of identification of devices.[19] Any information required under the FDCA must be prominently and conspicuously placed on a product's labeling so that an ordinary consumer would be likely to read and understand it.[20]

The FDA can subject certain types of labeling information to more stringent requirements. The use of established names provides an example. The secretary of the FDA may designate an official, or "established" name for a device in the interest of usefulness or simplicity.[21] If a device has an established name, that name must be printed prominently in type that is at least half as large as the type used for any proprietary name or designation for the device.[22] For restricted devices, this rule extends to advertisements and other descriptive printed material.[23]

Other mandatory disclosures are intended to promote the safe use of the device. Product labeling must include adequate directions for users, and adequate warnings against potentially hazardous misuse, or against unsafe dosage or methods or duration of use.[24] Labeling for devices subject to a performance standard may be required to prescribe the proper installation, maintenance, and operation of the device.[25] All advertisements and promotional material for restricted devices must include safety information consisting of a brief statement of the device's intended uses, relevant warnings, precautions, and side effects.[26] In special instances, where the secretary finds it necessary to protect public health, the FDA may require a full description of a device's components or formula, including the quantity of each ingredient.[27] In extraordinary circumstances, the secretary can even require prior approval of an ad's content.[28]

Finally, misbranding laws impose unique disclosure and monitoring obligations on producers and distributors of devices presenting a high risk of harm to users. Upon determining that a device presents an unreasonable risk of substantial harm to public health, the secretary may require a producer to issue notification of the risk to all prescribing health professionals.[29] Failure to issue the message renders the device misbranded. Similarly, the secretary may order a manufacturer to conduct post-market surveillance of the following types of class II or III devices: 1) those likely to have serious adverse health consequences upon failure; 2) those implanted in humans for more than a year; and 3) those that sustain or support life and are used outside of a controlled facility.[30] Devices that are not monitored in compliance with this provision are also deemed misbranded.

SUMMARY OF ADULTERATION REGULATIONS

Adulteration regulations are intended to ensure that marketed medical devices conform to FDA quality requirements. A device is considered adulterated if it is actually or potentially unclean or dangerous.[31] To safeguard against adulterated devices, the regulations address the conditions under which a device was manufactured, as well as its post-market condition.

A number of adulteration laws concern general safety issues. For example, the FDCA empowers the secretary to impose good manufacturing practice (GMP) requirements to ensure the safety and effectiveness of devices. The GMPs govern manufacturing, design validation, packing, storage, and installation of devices.[32] Nonconforming devices are considered adulterated. Similarly, devices that the FDA has banned are also adulterated.[33] Adulteration laws extend to product containers, which are adulterated if composed in whole or part of any poisonous or deleterious substance that may render the contents injurious to health.[34]

Some adulteration laws focus on the cleanliness of devices. A device is considered adulterated if it has any filthy, putrid, or decomposed substances.[35] Devices are also adulterated if they have been prepared, packed, or held under unsanitary conditions where they may have become filthy or rendered injurious to health.[36]

Other adulteration regulations address performance. The FDA enforces two types of performance standards: those established by the secretary, and those established by other organizations and recognized by the secretary. A device that is obligated to meet either of these standards will be considered adulterated if it does not conform to the standard in every respect.[37]

Class III devices are governed by a special set of adulteration regulations. They all relate to premarket approval requirements. If the device is subject to premarket approval, its producer must file both an application for premarket approval and a notice of completion of a product development protocol on time. If either submission is late, the device is deemed adulterated. The same result occurs when: 1) an application was filed and approval of the application has been denied, suspended, or withdrawn; 2) a notice was filed and declared incomplete; or 3) approval of the device under the protocol has been withdrawn.[38] If a device was originally classified as Class II and was then reclassified as Class III, it is considered adulterated if it does not have an effective, approved application for premarket approval, or if the application has been suspended or is otherwise ineffective.[39]

FDA INSPECTION

Statutory Authority to Conduct Establishment Inspections

Section 704 of the FDCA (21 USC. § 374) establishes the regulatory basis for an inspection of a device company. The Office of Regulatory Affairs is charged with enforcing the law. By way of background, the office's Web site is at www.fda.gov/ora/. The Web site also contains a link to all offices as well as contact information for each office: www.fda.gov/ora/inspect_ref/iom/iomoradir.html. Common resources are also listed at www.fda.gov/ora/inspect_ref/ default.htm. This page includes information provided to FDA investigators and inspectors to assist them in their daily activities. These are the highlights of the section:

- *Field management directives.* The primary vehicle for distributing procedural information/policy on the management of Office of Regulatory Affairs (ORA) field activities.

- *Guides to inspections of . . .* Guidance documents written to assist FDA personnel in applying FDA's regulations, policies, and procedures during specific types of inspection or for specific manufacturing processes.

- *IOM: Investigations Operations Manual. Updated: December, 2000.* Primary procedure manual for FDA personnel performing inspections and special investigations.

- *International Inspection Manual and Travel Guide.* Procedure manual for FDA personnel performing inspections and other FDA-related activities abroad.

- *Inspection technical guides.* Guidance documents that provide FDA personnel with technical background in a specific piece of equipment, or a specific manufacturing or laboratory procedure, or a specific inspectional technique, and so on.

- *Medical device GMP reference information.* www.fda.gov/cdrh/dsma/cgmphome.html.

Reasonableness of the Inspection. Investigators from the FDA are authorized to enter and to inspect facilities "at reasonable times and within reasonable limits and in a reasonable manner. . . ." [FDCA § 704(a)(1)(A), (B); 21 USC. § 374(a)(1)(A), (B)] Note that the only limitation is that the times and scope be "reasonable."

Frequency of Inspections. Establishments that manufacture restricted devices are subject to inspection pursuant to § 374 with a frequency of at least once in every successive two-year period, following a first inspection within two years of approval. [FDCA § 510(h); 21 USC. § 360(h)]

Consent Unnecessary. The authority to conduct an inspection is statutorily mandated by the FDCA. The inspection can be done without the consent of the owner, operator, or agent in charge of the inspection. *United States v. Del Camp Baking Mfg. Co.*, 345 F. Supp. 1371 (D. Del. 1972). Citing to: *U.S. v. Biswell*, 406 U.S. 311, 92 Sup. Ct. 1593 (1972). "When the officers asked to inspect respondent's locked storeroom, they were merely asserting their statutory right, and respondent was on notice as to their identity and the legal basis for their action. Respondent's submission to lawful authority and his decision to step aside and permit the inspection rather than face a criminal prosecution is analogous to a householder's acquiescence in a search pursuant to a warrant when the alternative is a possible criminal prosecution for refusing entry or a forcible entry. In neither case does the lawfulness of the search depend on consent; in both, there is lawful authority independent of the will of the householder who might, other things being equal, prefer no search at all. In this context, *Bumper v. North Carolina*, 391 U.S. 543, 88 Sup. Ct. 1788, 20 L. Ed. 2d 797 (1968), is inapposite, since there the police relied on a warrant that was never shown to be valid; because their demand for entry was not pursuant to lawful authority, the acquiescence of the householder was held an involuntary consent. In the context of a regulatory inspection system of business premises, which is carefully limited in time, place, and scope, the legality of the search depends not on consent but on the authority of a valid statute.

It is . . . apparent that if the law is to be properly enforced and inspection made effective, inspections without warrant must be deemed reasonable official conduct under the Fourth Amendment. . . . Here, if inspection is to be effective and serve as a credible deterrent, unannounced, even frequent, inspections are essential. In this context, the prerequisite of a warrant could easily frustrate inspection; and if the necessary flexibility as to time, scope, and frequency is to be preserved, the protections afforded by a warrant would be negligible."

A refusal to permit an inspection is a prohibited act and, therefore, punishable as a misdemeanor unless the investigator has failed to follow the procedures set forth in section 704 (that is, presenting of credentials and issuance of written Notice of Inspection) (FDCA § 304, 21 USC § 374).

Warrant Unnecessary. For the reasons that consent to an inspection is not necessary, a warrant likewise is not required. Warrantless inspections pursuant to section 704 of the FDCA are reasonable and do not violate the Fourth Amendment (FDCA § 704, 21 USC § 374). In reaching this conclusion, courts have considered the public health interest sought to be protected and that establishments operating in closely regulated industries, such as foods, drugs, cosmetics, and medical devices, voluntarily subject themselves to numerous government regulations and to the restrictions placed on such activity. As such, they have no reasonable expectation of privacy. *United States v. Jamieson-McKames Pharmaceuticals, Inc.*, 651 F. 2d 532 (8th Cir. 1981), *cert. denied* (1981); *Colonnade Catering Corp. v. United States*, 397 U.S. 72 (1970); *United States v. Biswell*, 406 U. S. 311 (1972).

Such warrantless searches are upheld because "when an entrepreneur embarks on such a business, he has chosen to subject himself to a full arsenal of governmental regulation," id. at 313, 98 Sup. Ct. at 1820 and "in effect consents to the restrictions placed on him." *Ibid*, citing *Almeida- Sanchez v. United States*, 413 U.S. 266, 271, 93 Sup. Ct. 2535, 2538, 37 L. Ed. 2d 596 (1973). Further, in the face of a long history of government scrutiny, such a proprietor has no "reasonable expectation of privacy." *Ibid*.

We think the drug manufacturing industry is properly within the Colonnade-Biswell exception to the warrant requirement. The drug manufacturing industry has a long history of supervision and inspection. The present Food, Drug, and Cosmetic Act has its origins in the Food and Drug Act of 1906, 34 Stat. 768. That act was an attempt by Congress "to exclude from interstate commerce impure and adulterated food and drugs" and to prevent the transport of such articles "from their place of manufacture." *McDermott v. Wisconsin*, 228 U.S. 115, 128, 33 Sup. Ct. 431, 433, 57 L. Ed. 754 (1913). *United States. v. Jamieson-McKames Pharmaceuticals, Inc.*, 651 F. 2d 532, 537 (8th Cir. 1981)

Likewise, giving warnings of constitutional rights to owners, operators, or agents in charge of establishments being inspected is not necessary. The issuance of Miranda warnings is not applicable when individuals are not in custody, which is the typical situation during FDA inspections. *United States v. Thriftimart, Inc.*, 429 F. 2d 1006 (9th Cir. 1970); *United States v. Jamieson-McKames Pharmaceuticals, Inc.*, 651 F. 2d 532 (8th Cir. 1981), *cert. denied* (1981).

Reasons for FDA Administrative Inspection

An inspection may occur for a variety of reasons. The earliest possible inspection is probably for the preapproval inspection. As a condition for the approval of the device, the FDA may inspect the company to determine its ability to produce the product as claimed, as well as its ability to comply with GMPs. Once the product has been approved, the company may also have an inspection as a part of the agency's routine or when it comes to the agency's attention that there may be violations of the act. Other types of enforcement actions taken by the agency, such as a seizure of a warning letter, might also trigger unannounced inspections. Likewise, if there has been a recall, the FDA might inspect a company to determine the background for the recall as well as to see what steps the company is taking to correct the problem. With an increasingly aware consuming public, the company might also expect to see inspections following consumer complaints.

A special enforcement initiative may be part of local or national initiatives and will focus on particular types of industries or products (for example, food warehouses, seafood processors, and drug products that are difficult to manufacture).

The Nuts and Bolts for Conducting Inspections

The *Investigation Operations Manual* is the basis for all inspections.[40] It outlines, in detail, the procedures that are followed by FDA investigators. The foreword to the manual notes:

> The *Investigations Operations Manual* (IOM) is the primary source of guidance regarding agency policy and procedures for field investigators and inspectors. This extends to all individuals who perform field investigation activities in support of the agency's public mission. Accordingly, it directs the conduct of all fundamental field investigational activities. Adherence to this manual is paramount to assure quality, consistency,

and efficiency in field operations. Although the IOM is the primary source of policy, the specific information in this manual is supplemented, not superseded, by other manuals and field guidance documents. Recognizing that this manual may not cover all situations or variables arising from field operations, any significant departures from IOM established procedures must have the concurrence of district management with appropriate documentation as needed.

Present Credentials and Notice of Inspection

Despite the fact that an inspection can be conducted without a warrant or consent, an inspection begins and an inspector can enter only "upon presenting appropriate credentials and a written Notice. . . ." The presentation of credentials and the written notice (FD Form 482) are to be presented to the owner, operator, or agent in charge of the facility.[41]

The policy requires that a separate notice of inspection is required for each inspection unless an investigator makes multiple entries during a single inspection continuing over a period of time.

Scope of Inspection

FDA investigators are authorized to enter any factory, warehouse, or establishment where devices are manufactured, processed, packed, or held before or after introduction into interstate commerce. Investigators are also authorized to enter any vehicle used to transport or hold these devices, or cosmetics, in interstate commerce. [FDCA § 704(a)(1)(A), 21 USC § 374(a)(1)(A)]

The FDA inspector can examine not only the premises but also all equipment, finished and unfinished materials, containers, and labeling within the establishment or vehicle in which the devices are manufactured, processed, packed, held, or transported. Copies of documents can also be made. The refusal to permit access or copying of required records is also a prohibited act [FDCA § 301(e), (f); 21 USC § 331(e), (f)] punishable as a misdemeanor.

There are limits, however. The agency's authority under the act does *not* extend to financial data, sales data (other than shipment data), pricing data, personnel data (other than data as to qualifications of technical and professional personnel performing functions subject to the act), or research data (other than data relating to devices and subject to reporting an inspection under regulations lawfully issued pursuant to sections 505(i) or (j), 507(d) or (g), 519, or 520(g), and data relating to other devices which in the case of a new drug would be subject to reporting or inspection under lawful regulations issued pursuant to section 505(j). [FDCA §§ 505(i), (j); 507(d), (g); 519; 520(g); 21 USC §§ 355(i), (j); 357(d), (g); 360i; 360j(g)]

FDA's Authority to Inspect Records of Interstate Shipment by Common Carriers and Recipients

Section 703 of the FDCA requires that, upon an inspector's request, carriers engaged in interstate commerce, as well as those who receive or hold devices, must permit access to and copying of all records showing the movement in interstate commerce of medical devices.

If requesting in writing, it is unlawful for any carrier or person to fail to permit access and copying of a record. Evidence obtained from a carrier or person receiving such articles pursuant to a written request is not to be used in a criminal prosecution of the person from whom such evidence was obtained. Common carriers are not subject to the other provisions of the FDCA merely by reason of their receipt, carriage, holding, or delivery of foods, drugs, devices, or cosmetics in the usual course of business as carriers. (FDCA § 703, 21 USC § 373)

If during the inspection the investigator obtains any sample of an article ("official sample"), a receipt describing the samples must be provided before the inspector leaves the premises. (FDCA § 704(c), 21 USC § 374(c); *see* Attachment 3, FD Form 484)

When an official sample is collected for analysis, the FDA must, upon request, provide a part of such official sample for examination or analysis to any person named on the label, to the owner, or to the owner's attorney or agent.[42]

Samples Taken During Inspection

Documentary Sample (DOC Sample). In addition to official samples, investigators may also collect DOC samples. DOC samples are collected in situations where an actual physical sample is not practical (for example, a large, permanently installed device), where a physical sample is no longer available, or where there is little need for laboratory examination. DOC samples might also include copies of labels and other documents subject to inspection such as transportation records, dealer affidavits, and an inventory of product on hand that documents the condition or practices at the facility or establishes facts of a past act.

301(k) Sample. A 301(k) sample is one collected from a product lot that became adulterated or misbranded while being held for sale after shipment in interstate commerce. Under section 301(k) of the FDCA, it is a prohibited act to do anything to a product after shipment in interstate commerce that results in the product being adulterated or misbranded. [FDCA § 301(k), 21 USC § 331(k)].

Post-Seizure Sample. After the U. S. marshal has seized a product, either the claimant or the government may obtain a sample for analysis. The sample may be collected only pursuant to court order. [FDCA § 304(c), 21 USC § 334(c)].

Investigational Sample (INV Sample). These samples are generally collected to document observations, support regulatory actions, or provide other information. INV samples may be used as evidence in court, and are sealed and handled by the FDA in a careful manner to protect their integrity. Examples of INV samples include:

- Raw materials in process and finished products to demonstrate manufacturing conditions

- Filth exhibits and other articles collected for exhibit purposes to demonstrate manufacturing or storage conditions

- Samples collected during reconditioning under a court decree to determine whether reconditioning was satisfactorily performed

- Survey samples to provide information about industry practices regarding a particular issue

- Complaint samples collected during investigation of an injury or illness

An *induced sample* is an official sample that is obtained by the FDA ordering by mail or through some other response to some type of advertisement or promotional activity. The sample is induced, generally by mail or telephone, without disclosing any association of the requestor or the transaction with the FDA.

In-Plant Photographs

Taking photographs during an inspection is not specifically authorized by the FDCA. Investigators, however, are directed to assume that they have authority to take photographs. The manual notes:

> Photos taken during establishment inspections are not classified as INV samples. They are exhibits. No C/R is used for photos taken unless the photos are part of an official sample. See *IOM 405* for information on official samples.
>
> Since photographs are one of the most effective and useful forms of evidence, every one should be taken with a purpose. Photographs should be related to unsanitary conditions contributing or likely to contribute filth to the finished product, or to practices likely to render it injurious or otherwise violative.

The manual continues:

> Do not request permission from management to take photographs during an inspection. Take your camera into the firm and use it as necessary just as you use other inspectional equipment.
>
> If management objects to taking photographs, explain that photos are an integral part of an inspection and present an accurate picture of plant conditions. Advise management the U.S. courts have held that photographs may lawfully be taken as part of an inspection.
>
> If management continues to refuse, provide them with the following references:
>
> 1. "*Dow Chemical v. United States*, 476 U.S. 227 (1986) This supreme court decision dealt with aerial photographs by EPA, but the court's language seems to address the right to take photographs by any regulatory agency. The decision reads in part, ". . . When Congress invests an agency with enforcement and investigatory authority, it is not necessary to identify explicitly each and every

technique that may be used in the course of executing the statutory mission. . . ."

2. *"United States of America v. Acri Wholesale Grocery Company, A Corporation, and Joseph D. Acri and Anthony Acri, Individuals,"* U.S. district court for southern district of Iowa. 409 F. Supp. 529. Decided February 24, 1976.

If management refuses, advise your supervisor so legal remedies may be sought to allow you to take photographs, if appropriate. If you have already taken some photos do not surrender film to management. Advise the firm it can obtain copies of the photos under the Freedom of Information Act. See *IOM 523.3.*

Affidavits and Interviews

The FDA may ask for an affidavit as a part of the inspection process. The purpose of an affidavit is to document shipment in interstate commerce of components or finished products. Affidavits may also be used to establish particular facts or individual responsibility that may later be used for enforcement purposes (seizure, injunction, and prosecution). There is no requirement in the FDCA, or elsewhere, for anyone to sign such an affidavit.

The FDCA does not expressly authorize investigators to interview a company's employees. However, discussions with company representatives may be useful or necessary during an inspection in order to provide an investigator with complete and accurate information in the event that the investigator may have questions or need an explanation of certain processes, procedures, or records. The facts and circumstances of a particular situation may influence the decision of whether to allow employee interviews.

The manual also recognizes that there may be some value to confidential interviews and establishes a protocol:

When you are faced with a situation involving informants who want to remain anonymous, contact your supervisor and follow the procedures here and any additional procedures in your district. It is particularly important that you take steps necessary to keep the identity confidential if your district concurs with this decision. When interviewing a confidential informant (CI) use the following procedures.

Type of meeting—Preference should be given to scheduling a personal interview with the CI rather than a telephone interview. At a face-to-face interview the investigator can assess the individual's demeanor, body language, overall presentation, and truthfulness.

Meeting location—The place and time of the interview should be the choice of the CI, unless there is a concern with personal safety. When the CI's suggested location is unsuitable, a good compromise could be a public meeting place such as a coffee shop. When a CI interview is conducted

> off FDA premises, notify your supervisor and/or colleagues of your destination, purpose, and estimated time of return. When an off-site interview has been completed, check in with your supervisor.
> *Interviewing methods/techniques*—CI interviews should be conducted by two investigators. The lead investigator conducts the interview while the second investigator takes notes and acts as a witness to the interview.

The Establishment Inspection Report

The report, called an establishment inspection report (EIR), is a detailed, written narrative that discusses the inspection. The EIR contains information such as the investigator's findings, history of the firm, persons interviewed, responsibility, operations, complaints, and corrective actions. It becomes the basis for the FDA's determination of what future action, if any, will be taken by the FDA. The reports are available under the Freedom of Information Act [Pub. L. No. 89-497, 80 Stat. 250 (1966), 5 USC. § 552 (1994)] if no action is contemplated.

After an Inspection

When an inspection is completed, the investigator is obligated to give to the owner, operator, or agent in charge a written report summarizing the findings of the inspection. [Inspectional Observations (FD 483)] The report identifies objectionable conditions or practices observed during the inspection. [FDCA § 704(b), 21 USC. § 374(b)]. (b) 21 USCA § 374 (b) Written report to owner; copy to secretary. Upon completion of any such inspection of a factory, warehouse, consulting laboratory, or other establishment, and prior to leaving the premises, the officer or employee making the inspection shall give to the owner, operator, or agent in charge a report in writing setting forth any conditions or practices observed by him which, in his judgment, indicate that any food, drug, device, or cosmetic in such establishment: 1) consists in whole or in part of any filthy, putrid, or decomposed substance; or 2) has been prepared, packed, or held under unsanitary conditions whereby it may have become contaminated with filth, or whereby it may have been rendered injurious to health. A copy of such report shall be sent promptly to the secretary. 21 USCA § 374 (b)

Before leaving the inspection, the investigator is required to meet with the company to discuss the results of the inspection. The manual notes:

> During the discussion, be frank, courteous, and responsive with management. Point out the observations listed on the FDA 483 are your observations of objectionable conditions found during the inspection, and explain the significance of each. Try to relate each listed condition to the applicable sections of the laws and regulations administered by the FDA. You should inform management during the closeout discussion the conditions listed may, after further review by the agency, be considered to be violations of the Food, Drug, and Cosmetic Act. Legal sanctions, including seizure, injunction, civil money penalties and prosecution, are available to FDA if establishments do not voluntarily correct serious conditions.

Thus, the primary purpose of such discussion is to inform management of the conditions observed by the investigator. Another purpose is to give the investigator an opportunity to elicit responses and commitments from the responsible individual. When the inspector's report is prepared there will be a discussion of the meeting.

Refusal to Permit Entry or Inspection or to Permit Access to or Copying of Records

If the owner, operator, or agent in charge refuses entry or inspection, the FDA's district office will approach either the Department of Justice and/or the local U.S. attorney's office to request assistance in obtaining an administrative inspection warrant from a federal magistrate judge.

The U.S. attorney's office and the FDA district office will work together in preparing an application for the warrant and present it to the judge or magistrate judge, who reviews it. If the application is found to be adequate, the magistrate judge will issue an administrative inspection warrant authorizing the FDA investigator to return to the facility and conduct the inspection.

If the owner, operator, or agent in charge still refuses entry or inspection pursuant to the warrant, that refusal is punishable as a contempt of court for that individual's failure to obey an order of a federal court. It is not unusual that such warrants of inspection would contain language that would allow the investigator broader inspectional authority (for example, the taking of photographs) than allowed under section 704.[43]

Notification, Replacement, and Recall: Overview

Under Section 518 (21 USC § 3605) of the FDCA, the FDA can issue three types of orders for resolving problems with medical devices.

Three main types of orders in ascending order of seriousness are:

- Notification

- Repair, replacement, or refund

- Recall

Note that separate provisions of the FDCA apply to electronic products. (21 USC § 360 11). Section 518 was originally included in the original Medical Device Amendments of 1976.[44] Since that time the sections has been amended twice.

The first change was in 1990 when the SMDA added subsection (e), which gave FDA explicit authority to order device recalls.[45] Two years later MDA modified the wording of the provision relating to repair, replacement, or refund, to make it easier for the FDA to take action.[46] The FDA has issued only one regulation that implements the recall provisions of section § 518(e).[47]

Notification Orders

If there is a problem with a medical device, the FDA might issue a notification order. The order will issue if the FDA determines that the device, "presents an unreasonable risk of substantial harm to the public health, that the notification will be necessary to eliminate the specific risk and that no more practical means is available to eliminate the risk." As provided by Section 518(a)[48]:

If the secretary determines that:

1. A device intended for human use that is introduced or delivered for introduction into interstate commerce for commercial distribution presents an unreasonable risk of substantial harm to the public health, and

2. Notification under this subsection is necessary to eliminate the unreasonable risk of such harm and no more practicable means is available under the provisions of this chapter (other than this section) to eliminate such risk, the secretary may issue such order as may be necessary to assure that adequate notification is provided in an appropriate form, by the persons and means best suited under the circumstances involved, to all health professionals who prescribe or use the device and to any other person (including manufacturers, importers, distributors, retailers, and device users) who should properly receive such notification in order to eliminate such risk. An order under this subsection shall require that the individuals subject to the risk with respect to which the order is to be issued be included in the persons to be notified of the risk unless the secretary determines that notice to such individuals would present a greater danger to the health of such individuals than no such notification. If the secretary makes such a determination with respect to such individuals, the order shall require that the health professionals who prescribe or use the device provide for the notification of the individuals whom the health professionals treated with the device of the risk presented by the device and of any action which may be taken by or on behalf of such individuals to eliminate or reduce such risk. Before issuing an order under this subsection, the secretary shall consult with the persons who are to give notice under the order.

Neither the statute nor any of the regulations define what constitutes "an unreasonable risk of substantial harm to public health." But a 1984 draft, "Medical Device Notification and Voluntary Safety Alert Guideline," defined the phrase to mean "actual or possible nonserious harm to a large number of persons as well as actual/or possible serious harm to a few individuals."

Unlike other orders under section 518, an "informal hearing" is not required before FDA issues an order under this section. But the statute directs that the secretary "shall consult with the persons who are to give notice under the order."

As a matter of practice, the FDA will notify the company and give it 10 days to consult with the FDA. The company then has the opportunity to negotiate the terms of the notification based upon the nature of the risk as well as the scope of the affected patient group.

The notice of the risk must be given either to the healthcare providers who prescribed the device or to the individuals who are users of the device. But if the FDA decides that the notification would present a greater danger to the health of such individuals, then "the order shall require that the health professionals who prescribe or use the device provide for the notification of the individuals whom the health professionals treated."

The statute uses the phrase "provide for the notification" rather than "notify" since individuals other than health professionals may be the appropriate persons to provide notification.[49] The FDA may also require notification of any other party, including manufacturers, importers, distributors, and device users, if it decides that the notification will help to eliminate the risk.

The content of the notification must be "in an appropriate form," and generally should include information about the risk and about any action which may be taken to eliminate or reduce the risk."

As a matter of procedure, the FDA relies on voluntary notifications called "safety alerts."[50] The 1984 Draft Guideline states that the purpose of the safety alert is to "inform health professionals and other appropriate persons of a situation that may present an unreasonable risk of substantial harm to the public health presented by a device in commercial distribution and intended for human use, in order to reduce or eliminate the risk."

The manufacturer can develop these without FDA comment, but as always, the FDA will consider the content and effectiveness of the alert to determine if any other notification should be ordered. If a company does issue a safety alert the FDA may classify it as a recall within the meaning of 21 CFR Part 7, as well as publish the alert as a recall in the weekly FDA Enforcement Report. These reports are archived at www.fda.gov/opacom/Enforce.html.

If the manufacturer issues a safety alert, the FDA requires that it review its efforts to ensure that the notification reached its intended audience.

The FDA has said that it will issue notification guidelines that include factors it will consider before ordering notifications under section 518(a). The guidelines may include a suggestion that manufacturers conduct focus testing of proposed notification letters to obtain initial patient feedback before issuing broader notification.

Between 1976 and 1992, the FDA did not use section 518(a). The FDA reported that in fiscal year 1992, the Recall and Notification Branch (RNB) of the Division of Compliance Operations II initiated 19 518(a) consultation letters and four 518(a) orders (Annual Report of the Office of Compliance and Surveillance Fiscal Year 1992).

Repair, Replacement, or Refund Orders

The next most serious regulatory power of dealing with a problem with a medical device is an order by the FDA that either directs the manufacturer to repair, refund, or replace the device.[51] The applicable statute is 21 USC § 360h(b), which was enacted in 1976 but has never been used. The procedure reveals the difficulties that the FDA would have if it were to take enforcement action under this section:

    b. Repair, replacement, or refund

        1. A. If, after affording opportunity for an informal hearing, the secretary determines that—

            (i) a device intended for human use that is introduced or delivered for introduction into interstate commerce for commercial distribution presents an unreasonable risk of substantial harm to the public health,

            (ii) there are reasonable grounds to believe that the device was not properly designed or manufactured with reference to the state of the art as it existed at the time of its design or manufacture,

(iii) there are reasonable grounds to believe that the unreasonable risk was not caused by failure of a person other than a manufacturer, importer, distributor, or retailer of the device to exercise due care in the installation, maintenance, repair, or use of the device, and

(iv) the notification authorized by subsection (a) of this section would not by itself be sufficient to eliminate the unreasonable risk and action described in paragraph (2) of this subsection is necessary to eliminate such risk, the secretary may order the manufacturer, importer, or any distributor of such device, or any combination of such persons, to submit to him within a reasonable time a plan for taking one or more of the actions described in paragraph (2). An order issued under the preceding sentence that is directed to more than one person shall specify which person may decide which action shall be taken under such plan and the person specified shall be the person who the secretary determines bears the principal, ultimate financial responsibility for action taken under the plan unless the secretary cannot determine who bears such responsibility or the secretary determines that the protection of the public health requires that such decision be made by a person (including a device user or health professional) other than the person he determines bears such responsibility.

B. The secretary shall approve a plan submitted pursuant to an order issued under subparagraph (A) unless he determines (after affording opportunity for an informal hearing) that the action or actions to be taken under the plan or the manner in which such action or actions are to be taken under the plan will not assure that the unreasonable risk with respect to which such order was issued will be eliminated. If the secretary disapproves a plan, he shall order a revised plan to be submitted to him within a reasonable time. If the secretary determines (after affording opportunity for an informal hearing) that the revised plan is unsatisfactory or if no revised plan or no initial plan has been submitted to the secretary within the prescribed time, the secretary shall (i) prescribe a plan to be carried out by the person or persons to whom the order issued under subparagraph (A) was directed, or (ii) after affording an opportunity for an informal hearing, by order prescribe a plan to be carried out by a person who is a manufacturer, importer, distributor, or retailer of the device with respect to which the order was issued but to whom the order under subparagraph (A) was not directed.

2. The actions that may be taken under a plan submitted under an order issued under paragraph (1) are as follows:

A. To repair the device so that it does not present the unreasonable risk of substantial harm with respect to which the order under paragraph (1) was issued.

B. To replace the device with a like or equivalent device that is in conformity with all applicable requirements of this chapter.

C. To refund the purchase price of the device (less a reasonable allowance for use if such device has been in the possession of the device user for one year or more—

    (i) at the time of notification ordered under subsection (a) of this section, or

    (ii) at the time the device user receives actual notice of the unreasonable risk with respect to which the order was issued under paragraph (1), whichever first occurs).

3. No charge shall be made to any person (other than a manufacturer, importer, distributor or retailer) for availing himself of any remedy, described in paragraph (2). and provided under an order issued under paragraph (1), and the person subject to the order shall reimburse each person (other than a manufacturer, importer, distributor, or retailer) who is entitled to such a remedy for any reasonable and foreseeable expenses actually incurred by such person in availing himself of such remedy.

Thus, before issuing an order under section 360h the FDA must first determine whether:

- The device presents an unreasonable risk of substantial harm to the public health.

- There are reasonable grounds to believe that the device was not properly designed or manufactured when the state of the art as it existed at the time of its design or manufacture is considered.

- There are reasonable grounds to believe that the risk is due to the conduct of the manufacturer, importer, distributor, or retailer and not due to improper installation, maintenance, repair, or use.

- Notification of the defect alone will not eliminate the risk, and that repair, replacement, or refund is necessary to eliminate the risk.

Congress intended 518(b) "to be in addition to and not as an alternative to the notification requirements."[52]

If the FDA were to decide that the defect is the type that requires it to invoke Section 518(b), it can direct the manufacturer, importer, distributor, or a combination of them to submit a plan for the repair, replacement, or refund of the device. If the FDA requires action from more than one party, it will designate which party has the responsibility to make the appropriate decisions for the plan. Once that party is designated, he or she is the one who will bear the financial responsibility for developing it and implementing it. However, the FDA does have the ability to revisit this assignment and make a new designation. The FDA also has the power to order a manufacturer, importer, distributor, or retailer of the device to reimburse any other manufacturer, importer, distributor, or retailer for expenses incurred in complying with the order. The only limitation is that the financial aspects of the order "shall not affect" any contractual agreements between the parties [FDCA § 518(c), 21 USC. § 360h(c)]. The FDA must also provide "opportunity for an informal hearing" before issuing the order requiring the plan.

Whoever has been designated by the FDA to develop the plan must have "a reasonable time" to submit a plan that satisfies the order. If a plan is not submitted, the FDA will then fashion one.

Depending on what the FDA orders, the plan must propose one of the following:

- Repair the device in a way that eliminates the specific risk

- Replace the device with a like or equivalent device that conforms to FDA requirements

- Refund the purchase price: either the full purchase price if the user has had the device for less than a year as of the time the user receives notice of the risk, or at a discounted purchase price if the user has had possession for one year or more

If the user repairs or replaces the device on its own as provided by the approved plan, the user can seek reimbursement of those reasonable and foreseeable expenses from whichever party is subject to the order.

The FDA must approve a submitted plan to ensure that it eliminates the unreasonable risk. Before a plan is rejected, the FDA must provide an opportunity for an informal hearing to review why it has been rejected. Upon disapproval, the FDA "shall order a revised plan to be submitted." If the FDA considers the revised plan to be unsatisfactory following opportunity for an informal hearing, the FDA shall prescribe one.

Again, largely because of the number of findings required and the elaborate procedures, the FDA has yet to issue an order under section 518(b).

RECALLS [FDCA § 518(E), 21 USC § 360H(E)]

Until the SMDA added Section 518(e), the FDA did not have explicit authority to order recalls of medical devices. Yet because the FDA never used its authority under 518(b), the recall authority added by Section 518(e) in 1990 provided a different kind of recall power. The FDA issued a final rule on mandatory recall procedures that became effective on May 17, 1997.

As described on the FDA Web site:

> Recalls are actions taken by a firm to remove a product from the market. Recalls may be conducted on a firm's own initiative, by FDA request, or by FDA order under statutory authority. A Class I recall is a situation in which there is a reasonable probability that the use of or exposure to a violative product will cause serious adverse health consequences or death. A Class II recall is a situation in which use of or exposure to a violative product may cause temporary or medically reversible adverse health consequences or where the probability of serious adverse health consequences is remote. A Class III recall is a situation in which use of or exposure to a violative product is not likely to cause adverse health consequences.[53]

The act defines "serious, adverse health consequences" to include "any significant adverse experience attributable to a device, including those which may be either life-threatening, or involve permanent or long-term injuries." (S. Rep. no. 513, 101st Cong., 2d Sess. 19 (1990).)The statutory and regulatory scheme provides for two types of recalls: the mandatory recall as well as a voluntary recall. The effect of the legislation is to provide the FDA with administrative injunctive power before there is a hearing extended to the company.

Mandatory Recall Order

The applicable regulations for a mandatory recall are set forth in 21 CFR Part 8. Under the regulation, before there is a recall, the FDA must find there is a reasonable probability that the device would cause serious, adverse health consequences or death. In such a case it will issue an order to cease distribution of a device and to notify healthcare professionals about the risk. For the purposes of the statute "reasonable probability" means "it is more likely than not that an event will occur." 31 CFR § 810.2(h)

Before it initiates a recall, the FDA will conduct a health hazard evaluation.[54] A health hazard evaluation is an evaluation by an ad hoc FDA committee that evaluates the risk and assigns a recall classification.

If the FDA decides that the device poses a risk, the order is directed to "the appropriate person," which may include manufacturers, importers, distributors, and retailers. The FDA then issues a two-part order to immediately cease distribution of the device and notify healthcare professionals as well as device user facilities. These groups are advised about the order and told to immediately stop using the device. The order will include the device's brand name; its common name; the model, catalog, or product code number; and other identifying information such as lot or serial numbers. It will also include a contact name at the agency.

As a matter of practice the FDA will provide an opportunity to consult with the agency before it issues a cease distribution and notification order.[55] The order identifies the specific device that is the subject of the order, the requirements of the order, and the basis for the recall.[56] The FDA may also include a model notification letter, which it considers binding on manufacturers, as well as a schedule for the completion of the notification.[57]

Once the order has been initiated, the FDA may require the manufacturer to provide specific information about the device that may include the number of devices that have been distributed, the names and addresses of all distributors, as well as the proposed strategy for complying with the order. The company can request a hearing on the actions required by the order. The company can also ask for a hearing to determine whether it should be modified, vacated, or amended to require a mandatory recall. The FDA can deny the request for a hearing if it determines that no genuine and substantial issue of fact is raised by the request. 21 CFR § 810.11(a). It can also submit a written request that the order be modified, vacated, or amended.[58] Normally there are three working days to request the hearing, but because of the seriousness of the action, the FDA may grant a shorter period. The hearing generally must be held between two to 10 working days after the FDA receives the request.[59] Once the hearing has been completed the FDA must provide a written notification of its final decision within 15 working days or 15 working days of the receipt of a written request for review of the order. 21 CFR §§ 810.11(e), (f), 810.12(c)

If there is a mandatory recall, the FDA will provide for notice to individuals who are subject to the device's risk. The FDA may seek to provide notice through the media if there are significant difficulties in identifying the group. The FDA also has the power to identify the scope the recall extends to (wholesale, retail, user), as well as a timetable for the recall. The FDA may require the manufacturer to use a model notification letter, to submit a proposed compliance strategy, and to give periodic progress reports.[60]

The only limitation to a recall is that the agency cannot order a recall if the health risks of recalling the device are greater than those of not recalling it.[61]

The notification must be by verified written communication that is conspicuously marked. Telephone calls or other personal contacts may be made in addition to, but are not a substitute for, the verified written communication.[62]

The notice may be provided through affected individuals' health professionals rather than directly to individuals if the FDA agrees this is appropriate and the most effective method of notification.[63]

Effectiveness checks for a recall are required, and a strategy must be submitted for approval.[64] The purpose of the effectiveness check is to ensure that the recall is working the way the plan intended. Follow-up communications must be sent to all who fail to respond to the initial communication.[65] The appropriate person can request termination of the order by certifying compliance and including a copy of the most current status report.[66]

The FDA may terminate the order after determining that the person named in the order has taken all reasonable notification efforts, and either removed or corrected the device.[67]

The FDA will publish new mandatory recalls in its weekly *FDA Enforcement Report* unless it determines that such notification will cause unnecessary and harmful anxiety in individuals, and that initial consultation between individuals and their health professionals is essential.

VOLUNTARY RECALLS

FDA Policy

Even when the statutory provisions under section 518 are not met, the FDA can request that a device be recalled, or a firm can recall a device on its initiative. The FDA often uses its powers to order a recall under section 518(e) as leverage in achieving voluntary recalls. The mechanics of a voluntary recall are set forth in 21 CFR Part 7 (which applies to all prescription products).

The FDA defines *recall* broadly as "a firm's removal or correction of a marketed product that the Food and Drug Administration considers to be in violation of the laws it administers and against which the agency would initiate legal action, for example, a seizure." Recalls do not include market withdrawals or stock recoveries, however.[68] And they are to be distinguished from a correction, which includes all changes in labeling, inspections, repairs, or adjustments to a device. If a correction is classified by the FDA as a recall, it will be publicized as such in the FDA enforcement report.

The FDA has posted its policies with respect to recalls that emphasize a collaborative effort between the agency and the company:

> The recall of a defective or possibly harmful consumer product often is highly publicized in newspapers and on news broadcasts. This is especially true when a recall involves foods, drugs, cosmetics, medical devices, and other products regulated by FDA.
>
> Despite this publicity, FDA's role in conducting a recall often is misunderstood not only by consumers, but also by the news media, and occasionally even by the regulated industry. The following headlines, which appeared in two major daily newspapers, are good examples of that misunderstanding: "FDA

Orders Peanut Butter Recall," and "FDA Orders 6,500 Cases of Red-Dyed Mints Recalled." The headlines are wrong in indicating that the Agency can "order" a recall. FDA has no authority under the Federal Food, Drug, and Cosmetic Act to order a recall, although it can request a firm to recall a product.

Most recalls of products regulated by FDA are carried out voluntarily by the manufacturers or distributors of the product. In some instances, a company discovers that one of its products is defective and recalls it entirely on its own. In others, FDA informs a company of findings that one of its products is defective and suggests or requests a recall. Usually, the company will comply; if it does not, then FDA can seek a court order authorizing the federal government to seize the product.

This cooperation between FDA and its regulated industries has proven over the years to be the quickest and most reliable method to remove potentially dangerous products from the market. This method has been successful because it is in the interest of FDA, as well as industry, to get unsafe and defective products out of consumer hands as soon as possible.

FDA has guidelines for companies to follow in recalling defective products that fall under the agency's jurisdiction. These guidelines make clear that FDA expects these firms to take full responsibility for product recalls, including follow-up checks to assure that recalls are successful.

Under the guidelines, companies are expected to notify FDA when recalls are started, to make progress reports to FDA on recalls, and to undertake recalls when asked to do so by the Agency.

The guidelines also call on manufacturers and distributors to develop contingency plans for product recalls that can be put into effect if and when needed. FDA's role under the guidelines is to monitor company recalls and assess the adequacy of a firm's action. After a recall is completed, FDA makes sure that the product is destroyed or suitably reconditioned and investigates why the product was defective.

Mechanics of a Recall

A manufacturer of any prescription product may voluntarily initiate a recall that is done "because manufacturers and distributors carry out their responsibility to protect the public health and well-being from products that present a risk of injury or gross deception or are otherwise defective." Sections 7.41 through 7.59 provide the guidance for the elements of a voluntary recall.

If a prescription product that has the potential to cause adverse health consequences appears to be in violation of the act, the firm should determine if the risk falls within a classification for a recall. These are:

1. Class I is a situation in which there is a reasonable probability that the use of, or exposure to, a violative product *will cause* serious adverse health consequences or death.

2. Class II is a situation in which use of, or exposure to, a violative product *may cause* temporary or medically reversible adverse health consequences *or where the probability of serious adverse health consequences is remote.*

3. Class III is a situation in which use of, or exposure to, a violative product is *not likely to cause* adverse health consequences.[69]

If the FDA becomes aware of this violation, it will engage in the same evaluation through an ad hoc committee of FDA scientists.[70] Factors that the committee as well as the firm should take into account when evaluating the nature of the risk and classification of the potential recall include:

1. Whether any disease or injuries have already occurred from the use of the product.

2. Whether any existing conditions could contribute to a clinical situation that could expose humans or animals to a health hazard. Any conclusion shall be supported as completely as possible by scientific documentation and/or statements that the conclusion is the opinion of the individual(s) making the health hazard determination.

3. Assessment of hazard to various segments of the population, for example, children, surgical patients, pets, livestock, and so on, who are expected to be exposed to the product being considered, with particular attention paid to the hazard to those individuals who may be at greatest risk.

4. Assessment of the degree of seriousness of the health hazard to which the populations at risk would be exposed.

5. Assessment of the likelihood of occurrence of the hazard.

6. Assessment of the consequences (immediate or long-range) of occurrence of the hazard.[71]

If it is found that there is a risk that warrants a recall, the firm either on its own or in conjunction with the FDA will create a recall strategy.

Recalls are to be used when "many lots of product have been widely distributed" and is an alternative to the seizure remedies available to the agency. Even though the FDA only has the power to order a recall for medical devices, it is not without alternatives if a company does not respond to its request:

> Seizure, multiple seizure, or other court action is indicated when a firm refuses to undertake a recall requested by the Food and Drug Administration, or where the agency has reason to believe that a recall would not be effective, determines that a recall is ineffective, or discovers that a violation is continuing.[72]

Alternatively, the FDA has the ability to suggest a recall if "a product that has been distributed presents a risk of illness or injury or gross consumer deception," the firm has not initiated a recall, and the FDA has determined that "agency action is necessary to protect the public health and welfare."[73]

If the FDA does request a recall, it will take these steps:

1. It will notify the firm of the determination and the need to begin a recall.

2. The notification must be made by letter or telegram, but this can be preceded by a oral communication or visit by an authorized representative followed by written confirmation.

3. The notification in whatever form must identify the nature of the violation, the classification of the health hazard, the recall strategy, and other "appropriate instructions."

If the firm agrees with the FDA evaluation, it can follow up with its input for the need for the recall or how it should be conducted.[74] The FDA also has the ability to tell the firm that, in its opinion, the product violates the law and not request a recall. In such a situation the firm may decide on its own to initiate a recall that is then governed by 21 CFR 7.46 governing firm-initiated recalls.[75]

If the reason for the removal or correction is not apparent, the firm should consult with the appropriate FDC district office. In the words of the regulation, such consultation should occur when "the reason for the removal or correction is not obvious or clearly understood but where it is apparent, for example, because of complaints or adverse reactions regarding the product, that the product is deficient in some respect."[76]

The firm can initiate the recall if it "believes the product to be violative." If it does so, it must notify the appropriate district office identified in the regulations (Section 5.115). "Such removal or correction will be considered a recall only if the Food and Drug Administration regards the product as involving a violation that is subject to legal action, for example, seizure."[77]

Once this decision is made, the firm must provide the FDA with the following information:

1. Identity of the product involved

2. Reason for the removal or correction and the date and circumstances under which the product deficiency or possible deficiency was discovered

3. Evaluation of the risk associated with the deficiency or possible deficiency

4. Total amount of such products produced and/or the time span of the production

5. Total amount of such products estimated to be in distribution channels

6. Distribution information, including the number of direct accounts and, where necessary, the identity of the direct accounts

7. A copy of the firm's recall communication if any has issued, or a proposed communication if none has issued

8. Proposed strategy for conducting the recall

9. Name and telephone number of the firm official who should be contacted concerning the recall[78]

The FDA then reviews the materials and conducts its own investigation to decide upon the classification of the recall as well as modifications to the suggested strategy (discussed later). The FDA also advises the firm that the recall will be placed in the weekly FDA enforcement report.

If there is a firm-initiated recall, the FDA remains involved:

These sections also recognize that recall is an alternative to a Food and Drug Administration–initiated court action for removing or correcting violative, distributed products by setting forth specific recall procedures for the Food and Drug Administration to monitor recalls and assess the adequacy of a firm's efforts in recall.

RECALL STRATEGY

Overview

The recall strategy is defined by the regulations to be a planned specific course of action to be taken in conducting a specific recall, which addresses the depth of recall, need for public warnings, and extent of effectiveness checks for the recall.[79]

The strategy is shaped by these factors:

1. Results of health hazard evaluation

2. Ease in identifying the product

3. Degree to which the product's deficiency is obvious to the consumer or user

4. Degree to which the product remains unused in the marketplace

5. Continued availability of essential products[80]

While the FDA will review the adequacy of a strategy, the firm is encouraged not to delay its recall while waiting for FDA.[81]

ELEMENTS OF A RECALL STRATEGY

The regulations provide the following elements of a recall strategy.

Depth of Recall

The individuals and entities to which a recall should be directed are dependent upon two factors: the seriousness of the risk and the scope of the distribution chain. The levels that must be addressed include:

1. Consumer or user level, which may vary with product, including any intermediate wholesale or retail level

2. Retail level, including any intermediate wholesale level

3. Wholesale level[82]

The regulations are also very clear as to the obligations and content of communications with those who are being asked to return the prescription product, again all of it dependent upon the seriousness of the hazard involved. The purpose of the communication, whatever its form, should be:

1. That the product . . . is subject to a recall

2. That further distribution or use of any remaining product should cease immediately

3. Where appropriate, that the direct account should in turn notify its customers who received the product about the recall

4. Instructions regarding what to do with the product[83]

The communication can be sent by telegram, mailgram, or first-class letter.

The document should be "conspicuously marked, preferably in bold red type, on the letter and the envelope" that the matter involves a recall. "The letter and the envelope should be also marked: "urgent" for class I and class II recalls and, when appropriate, for class III recalls. Telephone calls or other personal contacts should ordinarily be confirmed by one of the aforementioned methods and/or documented in an appropriate manner."[84]

The regulations also provide what the contents of the letter should include:

1. Be brief and to the point.

2. Identify clearly the product, size, lot number(s), code(s) or serial number(s), and any other pertinent descriptive information to enable accurate and immediate identification of the product.

3. Explain concisely the reason for the recall and the hazard involved, if any.

4. Provide specific instructions on what should be done with respect to the recalled products.

5. Provide a ready means for the recipient of the communication to report to the recalling firm whether it has any of the product, for example, by sending a postage-paid, self-addressed postcard or by allowing the recipient to place a collect call to the recalling firm.[85]

They also detail what should not be included:

2. The recall communication should not contain irrelevant qualifications, promotional materials, or any other statement that may detract from the message.[86]

The firm should also develop a follow-up strategy for those who do not respond.

Public Warning

The second component of the recall strategy is to address the issue of how the public is to be alerted about the recall. It is limited to "urgent situations where other means for preventing use of the recalled product appear inadequate."

The regulations make clear that the preference is for the FDA to work with the firm and to have the agency issue the publicity. If the firm decides to issue its own warning, the FDA suggests that it give the agency the opportunity to comment upon its content. The regulations continue:

The recall strategy will specify whether a public warning is needed and whether it will issue as:

1. General public warning through the general news media, either national or local as appropriate

2. Public warning through specialized news media, for example, professional or trade press, or to specific segments of the population such as physicians, hospitals, and so on[87]

Section 7.50 emphasizes that the FDA will advise the public of the recall in its weekly enforcement report.[88]

Effectiveness Checks

A recall is only as good as its effectiveness in getting a return of the device. Key to planning a recall is developing a plan for a follow-up with those who have been contacted by the notification. As noted by the regulations: "The purpose of effectiveness checks is to verify that all consignees at the recall depth specified by the strategy have received notification about the recall and have taken appropriate action."

The regulations emphasize that the contacts can take a variety of methods that include "personal visits, telephone calls, letters, or a combination thereof." The regulations also emphasize that while the firm is ultimately responsible for conducting the checks, the FDA will assist "where necessary and appropriate."

Depending upon the classification of the risk, the recall strategy must also include the percentage of individuals to be contacted:

1. Level A: 100 percent of the total number of consignees to be contacted

2. Level B: Some percentage of the total number of consignees to be contacted, which percentage is to be determined on a case-by-case basis, but is greater that 10 percent and less than 100 percent of the total number of consignees

3. Level C: 10 percent of the total number of consignees to be contacted

4. Level D: 2 percent of the total number of consignees to be contacted

5. Level E: No effectiveness checks[89]

Status Reports

As a part of the recall process, the firm must develop a plan to submit periodic status reports to the appropriate district office to assist the agency in evaluating the progress of the recall.[90] The FDA will decide the frequency of the reports depending upon the urgency of the recall, which will range from two to four weeks. The reports should include the following:

1. Number of consignees notified of the recall, and date and method of notification

2. Number of consignees responding to the recall communication and quantity of products on hand at the time it was received

3. Number of consignees who did not respond

4. Number of products returned or corrected by each consignee contacted and the quantity of products accounted for

5. Number and results of effectiveness checks that were made

6. Estimated time frames for completion of the recall 21 CFR 7.53(b)

   The reports end only when the recall is terminated.[91]

Termination of the Recall

Once the FDA decides that "all reasonable efforts have been made to remove or correct the product in accordance with the recall strategy, and when it is reasonable to assume that the product subject to the recall has been removed and proper disposition or correction has been made commensurate with the degree of hazard of the recalled product," it will give written notification to the firm. Likewise the firm can request in writing with its current status report that the recall be terminated for the same reasons.[92]

Court-Ordered Recalls: Initiated by the FDA Seeking Injunctive Relief

The courts were initially hesitant to become involved with recalls but are now more willing to do so to balance the extent of danger to the public as opposed to the harm to the manufacturer if there is a recall.

And example is *United States v. K-N Enterprises*, 461 F. Supp. 988 (N.D. Ill 1978) that held (as noted in the case summary):

> Government filed motion for preliminary injunction and temporary restraining order seeking recall and prohibition against the manufacture of certain drugs and certain devices pursuant to Federal Food, Drug and Cosmetic Act. The district court, held that: 1) upon showing that one drug was "misbranded" under act and that another drug had not been approved by Food and Drug Administration before introduction into interstate commerce, and upon conclusions that government would be likely to prevail on those issues, that harm which might be inflicted upon the public by continued distribution of those drugs greatly outweighed possible damage inflicted upon defendants, and that government had no adequate remedy at law, preliminary injunction pendente lite would issue requiring recall of drugs and prohibiting their further distribution or manufacture; and 2) absent finding that government had reasonable likelihood of prevailing on the merits of its claim that devices in question violated act, preliminary injunction would not be issued as to distribution or manufacture of those devices.

United States v. Lanpar Company, 293 F. Supp. 147 (N.D. Tx 1968) is an example of what a court can do even if the FDA can't order a recall.

The court ruled that the United States was entitled to an injunction restraining and enjoining the manufacturer as follows:

1. From introducing or causing to be introduced into interstate commerce any of the products until the method used in, and the facilities and controls used for, their manufacture, processing, packaging and holding conform to and are operated and administered in conformity with current good manufacturing practices to assure that such products meet the requirements of the act as to safety and have the identity and strength and meet the quality and purity characteristics which they purport or are represented to possess. This order will be suspended for ninety days in order to afford Lanpar Company a reasonable time to bring their manufacturing practices into conformity with current good manufacturing practices by correcting the deficiencies outlined in paragraphs VI and VIII of the findings.

2. From causing any of the drugs to be accompanied by the following written, printed and graphic matter; Lanpar technical reports and bulletins; Lanpar clinical reviews, and leaflets, which have previously been sent to physicians. In this connection, Lanpar shall recall and destroy all such reviews, reports, bulletins, and leaflets previously sent to customers.

3. From writing, printing, distributing, or causing to be distributed any written, printed, or graphic matter or any other written, printed, or graphic matter which contains statements which represent and suggest that any of said drugs, singly or in combination are safe and effective in

the treatment of hyperthyroidism, amenorrhea and hypomenorrhea; can safely bring about weight loss without the benefit of rigid dieting; that obesity is usually a disorder of metabolism and that use of said drugs will cause a change toward the normal metabolism; that obesity is most commonly due to a derangement and disturbance of gland system synchronous function, since each gland must work in harmonious collaboration with the other endocrine glands in order to produce perfect functional balancing and that obesity results when faulty secretions interfere with the proper utilization of stored fats; that if the gastrointestinal and glandular balance were perfect, weight would be normal, that digitalis safely and satisfactorily curtails hunger and appetite and is practically devoid of untoward results; and that said drugs are safe and effective adjuncts in the treatment of all obesity; which statements are false and misleading since said drugs are not safe and effective for such purposes, and since the statements are otherwise contrary to fact.

4. From causing Thyalis or any combination of thyroid and digitalis to be sold or delivered in interstate commerce. In this connection Lanpar is ordered to have all drugs containing a combination of thyroid and digitalis returned and destroyed.

5. From causing digitalis to be sold or delivered in interstate commerce for the treatment of obesity or if Lanpar has reason to believe such drug will be used in the treatment of obesity.

6. Lanpar is directed to reword labels on bottles so as to include the following:

   a. On all bottles of digitalis: 'Warning: Not to be used for obesity. The administration of digitalis may induce digitalis toxicity. The manifestations of digitalis toxicity include loss of appetite, nausea, vomiting, diarrhea, abdominal pain, abnormalities of vision, and abnormal rhythms of the heart. Any side effect should immediately be called to your physician's attention. 'Dosage—as prescribed by physician.

   b. On all bottles of thyroid drugs: 'Warning: Not to be used in hyperthyroid patients for the treatment of obesity. Excessive administration of thyroid may induce an excessive amount of circulating thyroid hormone in the body and may reproduce, essentially, a disease called hyperthyroidism which may be manifested by increased metabolic rate, accelerated circulation, increased pulse pressure, loss of weight, nervousness, tremor, aberrations in reproductive function, and irregularities in heart rhythm. Any side effect should immediately be called to your physician's attention.' Dosage—as prescribed by physician.

United States v. Lit Drug Company, 333 F. Supp. 990 (D.N.J. 1971)—other ways to effect a recall—make sure that it never gets out. In this case involving a variety of prescription medicines including reserpine and digitalis courts have ordered that:

First, the methods, facilities and controls for manufacturing, processing, packaging, and labeling of defendants' drugs were to be brought in conformity with the current good manufacturing practices, as defined in 21 C.F.R. S 133.1-14. Defendants were directed to correct ten deficient practices in their quality control and record keeping.

As a second condition upon future interstate commerce, defendants were required to grant duly authorized Food and Drug Administration inspectors access to defendants' plant for the purpose of inspecting defendants' records, materials, equipment, and labeling in order to insure, to the satisfaction of the government, that defendants had in fact realigned the operation of the plant in conformity with current good manufacturing practices.

Third, all the drugs on hand at defendants' plant site were to be subject to examination by officials of the Food and Drug Administration, assays were to be made in order to assure the safety, identity, purity, strength, and quality of these drugs, and recalls were to be made of any line of drug determined to be adulterated or misbranded. These drugs would then likewise be examined and, if similarly defective, destroyed or brought into compliance with the law under the supervision of the Food and Drug Administration. The expenses for the inspecting, assaying, and recall operations were to be borne by the defendants.

Recall Web Sites

Helpful Web sites include:

- Recalls and safety alerts: www.fda.gov/opacom/7alerts.html.

- Enforcement reports: www.fda.gov/opacom/Enforce.html. A weekly publication that contains information on actions taken in connection with agency regulatory activities, such as recalls and field corrections, medical device notification, injunctions, seizures, prosecutions, and indictments.

- Medical product safety information: www.fda.gov/medwatch/safety.html. Provides links to medical device reporting data files, adverse drug reaction reporting data files, labeling changes related to drug safety, annual adverse drug experience report, "dear health professional letters," and other safety notifications.

- Medical device safety alerts, public health advisories, and notices: www.fda.gov/cdrh/safety.html (maintained by the Center for Devices and Radiological Health).

- Recalls and market withdrawals of fractionated blood and plasma products: www.fda.gov/cber/recalls.html (maintained by the Center for Biologics Evaluation and Research).

- Recalls: FDA, Industry Cooperate to Protect Consumers: www.fda.gov/fdac/features/895_recalls.html.

- A four-page article from the October 1995 issue of *FDA Consumer* magazine.

☐ **Endnotes** ☐

1. 21 USC. §321(h) (Pub. L. 94-295, §3(a)(1)(A).
2. Id.
3. 21 USC §360i; Publ L. 94-295 §6(a).
4. 21 USC §360aaa-aaa-1 (2001).
5. 21 USC §360bbb (2001).
6. 21 USC §§1-15 (1934) [repealed in 1938 by 21 U.S.C. §392(a)].
7. 21 USC §§352(o), 360(j) (2001).
8. 21 USC §§352(b), 352(0) (2001).
9. 21 USC §§352(o), 360(b) (2001).
10. 21 USC §§352(o), 360(j) (2001).
11. 21 USC §§352(o), 360(k), 360d, 360e (2001).
12. 21 USC §§352(a), 352(q) (2001).
13. 21 USC §352(j) (2001).
14. 21 USC §352(q) (2001).
15. 21 USC §60(j)(1)(B)(ii) (2001). The FDCA distinguishes between "label" and "labeling." A "label" refers to written, printed, or graphic statements that appear upon "the immediate container" of an article. "Labeling" encompasses all labels, as well as additional written, printed, or graphic statements appearing upon any container or wrapper for the article, the article itself, or any material accompanying the article.
16. 21 USC §360(j)(1)(A), 360(j)(1)(B)(i) (2001).
17. 21 USC §360(j)(1)(A) (2001).
18. 21 USC §352(b) (2001).
19. 21 USC §§352(b), 352(0), 360(e) (2001).
20. 21 USC §352(c) (2001).
21. 21 USC §358 (2001).
22. 21 USC §352(e)(2) (2001).
23. 21 USC §352(r) (2001).
24. 21 USC §352(f) (2001).
25. 21 USC §§352(s), 260d(2)(C) (2001).
26. 21 USC §352(r) (2001).
27. Id.
28. Id.
29. 21 USC §§352(t), 360h (2001).
30. 21 USC §§352(t), 360l (2001).
31. 21 USC §351(a)(1) (2001).
32. 21 USC §351(h) (2001).
33. 21 USC §360(j)(1)(A) (2001).
34. 21 USC §351(a)(3) (2001).
35. Id.
36. 21 USC §351(a)(2)(A) (2001).
37. 21 USC §351(e)(1)-(2) (2001).
38. 21 USC §351(f)(1)(A)(i)-(ii) (2001).
39. 21 USC §§351(f)(1)(B)(i)-(ii); 351(f)(1)(C) (2001).
40. The full manual can be found at www.fda.gov/ora/inspect_ref/iom/default.htm
41. A sample form can be found at www.fda.gov/ora/inspect_ref/iom/exhibits/x510a.pdf
42. FDCA § 702(b), 21 USC § 372(b).
43. FDCA § 74, 21 USC § 374.
44. MDA, Pub. L. No. 94-295, 90 Stat. 539 (1976), codified at 15 USC. § 55 (1994); 21 USC §§301, 331, 334, 351, 352, 358, 360, 374, 379, 381.

45. Pub. L. No. 101-629, 104 Stat. 4511 (1990), codified at 21 USC. §§ 301 note, 321, 333, 333 note, 351, 353, 360, 360c, 360c note, 360d-i, 360i notes, 360j, 360j note, 3601, 360gg-hh, 360hh note, 360ii-ss, 383, 383 note; 42 USC §§ 263b-n (Supp. 1991).
46. Pub. L. No. 102-300, 106 Stat. 238 (1992), 21 USC §§ 301 note, 321, 331, 334, 346a, 352, 353, 356, 357, 360c-d, 371, 372, 372a, 376, 381; 42 USC §§ 262.
47. *See* 21 CFR pt. 810 (effective May 19, 1997).
48. FDCA § 518(a), 21 USC § 360h(a).
49. *H.R. Cong. Rep. No.* 1090, 94th Cong. 60, 2nd Sess. (1976)(reprinted in 1976 U.S.C.C.A.N. 1112-13).
50. FDA 's site posts safety alerts that can be used to develop sample forms. www.fda.gov/cdrh/safety.html. An individual can also subscribe to e-mail notification through the Web site.
51. FDCA §518(b), (c), 21 USC §360h(b), (c)
52. *H.R. Rep. No.* 953, 94th Cong., 2nd Sess. (1976).
53. By "serious, adverse health consequences," Congress meant "any significant adverse experience attributable to a device, including those which may be either life-threatening, or involve permanent or long-term injuries, but excluding those non-life-threatening injuries that are temporary and reasonably reversible" [*S. Rep. No.* 513, 101st Cong., 2nd Sess. (1990)].
54. See 61 Fed. Reg. 59,004, 59,005 (1996).
55. 21 CFR § 810.10(a).
56. 21 CFR § 810.10(b).
57. 21 CFR § 810.10(c).
58. 21 CFR §§ 810.10(e), (f); 810.11(b).
59. 21 CFR §§ 810.11 (a), (e).
60. 21 CFR §§ 810.13(b), (d); 810.14.
61. FDCA § 518(e) (2) (B) (i) (I), (II); 21 USC § 360h(e) (2) (B) (i) (I), (II).
62. 21 CFR § 810.15(b).
63. 21 CFR § 810.14(C)(2).
64. 21 CFR § 810.14(C)(3).
65. 21 CFR § 810.15(d).
66. 21 CFR § 810.17(a).
67. 21 CFR § 810.17(b).
68. 21 CFR § 7.3(g).
69. 21 CFR § 7.3(m).
70. 21 CFR § 7.41.
71. 21 CFR § 7.41(a).
72. 21 CFR § 7.40(c).
73. 21 USC § 7.45.
74. 21 CFR § 7.45.
75. 21 CFR § 7.46(b).
76. 21 CFR § 7.48(d).
77. 21 CFR § 7.46.
78. 21 CFR § 7.46(a).
79. 21 CFR § 7.3.
80. 21 CFR § 7.42(a)(1).
81. 21 CFR § 7.42(a)(2).
82. 21 CFR § 7.42(a)(1).
83. 21 CFR § 7.49(a).
84. 21 CFR § 7.49(b).
85. 21 CFR § 7.49(c).

86. 21 CFR § 7.49(c).
87. 21 CFR § 7.42(b)(2).
88. 21 CFR § 7.50.
89. 21 CFR § 7.42(b)(3).
90. 21 CFR § 7.53.
91. 21 CFR § 7.53(c).
92. 21 CFR § 7.55.

Chapter 2

U.S. Regulation

QUALITY SYSTEM REGULATION

The quality system regulation published in 1996 was a revision of the medical device good manufacturing practice regulation. The following sections provide detail and guidance on each section of the regulation. The sections are intended to be brief overviews and not extensive evaluations of the regulation. Each section contains an overview, excerpts from the regulation itself, and a discussion. The reader should refer to the regulation (21CFR 820) and the preamble as published in the Federal Register.

PREAMBLE

The preamble was published in the Federal Register/vol. 61/no. 195 October 7, 1996 and precedes *Part 820 Quality System Regulation for Medical Devices.* The preamble also includes changes to *21 CFR Part 808 Exemptions from Federal Preemption of State and Local Medical Device Requirements* and *21 CFR 812 Investigational Device Exemptions.* The FDA's rationale for the quality system regulation, as it is presently written, is contained in the preamble. The information is a valuable resource for interpretation and provides insight into the position the FDA has taken in stating the requirements.

The preamble is organized in the following manner:

Supplementary Information:

I	Background
II	Decision to Make Working Draft Available for Comment
III	Open Public Meeting and GMP Advisory Committee
IV	Implementation of the Final Rule
V	Response to Comments and Rationale for Changes
VI	Summary of Changes from the July 1995 Working Draft to the Final Rule and Rationale
VII	Environmental Impact

Discussion

Section I discusses the background for the 1996 version of the quality system regulation identifying the SMDA, which provided the FDA clear authority to amend the FD&C Act section 510(f) adding preproduction design controls to the current good manufacturing practice (cGMP) regulation.

Sections II and III provide historical information as to how the FDA solicited feedback on the 1993 medical devices; cGMP regulations; proposed revisions; request for comments. The subsequent publication of the *1995 Working Draft* incorporated the FDA's response to the comments and allowed a final review period before issuing the final regulation October 7, 1996.

Section IV provides the rationale for the implementation of the final rule in two phases, where the FDA implemented a special one-year transition program, which allowed manufacturers a grace period to become fully compliant with the requirements of § 820.30 Design Controls. This section emphasizes that manufacturers were responsible to take reasonable steps to come into compliance with the requirements during the June 1, 1997 to June 1, 1998 period. The FDA stated that firms would be inspected against the design control requirements during the transition period, but a separate design control inspection strategy report would be issued in lieu of an FDA Form 483 for observed noncompliances.

Of primary importance in understanding the content of the quality system regulation is Section V Response to Comments and Rationale for Changes. The FDA's response to the working draft, as well as explanations for changes, is contained in 204 comments that cover the entire scope of the quality system regulation, subparts A through O. The FDA conveys its support for international harmonization of standards governing medical devices and provides rationale for not adopting ISO 9001:1994 verbatim. Complications with copyrights issues were a first concern and secondly, the FDA's position that ISO 9001:1994 as a quality system standard is insufficient to protect the public health. Throughout this section of the preamble the FDA makes reference to the ISO 9001:1994 standard and ISO 13485 and provides specific rationale for similarities or differences relevant to the subpart or requirement discussed.

Section VII Environmental Impact states that an environmental impact statement is not required, as the final rule does not have a significant impact on the human environment.

The economic impact discussed in Section IX summarizes that changes to the cGMP regulation will require manufacturers engaged in design, manufacture, contract sterilization, and packaging of medical devices to expand their quality systems to include new areas such as preproduction quality assurance and purchasing controls. This section includes comments from the 1993 proposed changes to the cGMP regulation and the FDA's supporting rationale for changes to the regulation emphasizing close harmonization with ISO standards where possible.

Section X Congressional Review identifies the changes required to be considered a major rule and is followed by specific changes to the following sections: *Part 808—Exemptions from Federal Preemption of State and Local Medical Device Requirements; Part*

812—Investigational Device Exemptions; and a complete rewrite of *Part 820—Quality System Regulation for Medical Devices.*

SCOPE

The purpose of the scope is to state that the requirements in Part 820 regulate the methods, facilities, and controls used for the design, manufacture, packaging, labeling, storage, installation, and servicing of all finished devices intended for human use. The regulation is intended to ensure that finished devices are safe and effective and otherwise in compliance with the FDCA. Part 820 establishes the fundamental requirements applicable to manufacturers of finished devices, and clarifies where manufactures that engage in only some operations of the part need only to comply with those requirements applicable to their operations.

The regulation is broad in that it applies to a variety of medical devices, and the implementation of the requirements will vary based on the size of the organization, the complexity of the medical device, and the risks associated with the product.

The following section will address the individual regulatory requirement referencing the section of the quality system regulation, applicable definitions, and important points following the section.

Regulatory Requirement 21 CFR § 820.1(a) Applicability

1. Current good manufacturing practice (cGMP) requirements are set forth in this quality system regulation. The requirements in this part govern the methods used in, and the facilities and controls used for, the design, manufacture, packaging, labeling, storage, installation, and servicing of all finished devices intended for human use. The requirements in this part are intended to ensure that finished devices will be safe and effective and otherwise in compliance with the Federal Food, Drug, and Cosmetic Act (the act). This part establishes basic requirements applicable to manufacturers of finished medical devices. If a manufacturer engages in only some operations subject to the requirements in this part, and not in others, that manufacturer need only comply with those requirements applicable to the operations in which it is engaged. With respect to class I devices, design controls apply only to those devices listed in 21 CFR § 820.30(a)(2). This regulation does not apply to manufacturers of components or parts of finished devices, but such manufacturers are encouraged to use appropriate provisions of this regulation as guidance. Manufacturers of human blood and blood components are not subject to this part, but are subject to part 606 of this chapter.

2. The provisions of this part shall be applicable to any finished device as defined in this part, intended for human use, that is manufactured, imported, or offered for import in any state or territory of the United States, the District of Columbia, or the Commonwealth of Puerto Rico.

3. In this regulation the term "where appropriate" is used several times. When a requirement is qualified by "where appropriate," it is deemed to be "appropriate" unless the manufacturer can document justification otherwise. A requirement is "appropriate" if nonimplementation could reasonably be expected to result in the product not meeting its specified requirements or the manufacturer not being able to carry out any necessary corrective action.

Discussion

The regulations apply to manufacturers of finished medical devices that are intended for human use, which are manufactured, imported, or offered for import, in any state or territory of the United States, the District of Columbia, or the Commonwealth of Puerto Rico. Manufacturers of blood and blood components are not subject to 21 CFR Part 820, but rather 21 CFR Part 606. Component manufacturers are not subject to the requirements of this part, but are encouraged to comply with the regulation as guidance. Finished device manufacturers are responsible under § 820.50 Purchasing controls to ensure that component manufacturers (namely suppliers) meet specified requirements.

The term *manufacturer* is defined in section § 820.3(o) and includes people who perform some or all of the functions identified. It is important to recognize that while a firm may not be involved in all functions necessary from design to distribution, they may likely be considered a manufacturer under this regulation and be required to comply with the requirements applicable to their operation.

Several requirements are qualified with the term *where appropriate* throughout 21 CFR Part 820. When a requirement has been identified as "where appropriate," it is to be considered appropriate if nonimplementation may contribute to the product not meeting specified requirements, or if the manufacturer's ability to facilitate or carry out corrective action may be compromised as a result of not implementing the requirement. Objective evidence, including a firm's rationale, must be documented when a "where appropriate" requirement has not been implemented.

Regulatory Requirement 21 CFR § 820.1(b) Limitations

The quality system regulation in this part supplements regulations in other parts of this chapter except where explicitly stated otherwise. In the event that it is impossible to comply with all applicable regulations, both in this part and in other parts of this chapter, the regulations specifically applicable to the device in question shall supersede any other generally applicable requirements.

Discussion

The quality system regulation applies to all medical devices unless stated otherwise. Certain class I devices have been exempted from the design control requirements, while the reclassification of other devices may identify certain products that are exempt from specific sections of this regulation.

Regulatory Requirement 21 CFR § 820.1(c) Authority

Part 820 is established and issued under authority of sections 501, 502, 510, 513, 514, 515, 518, 519, 520, 522, 701, 704, 801, 803 of the act (21 USC 351, 352, 360, 360c, 360d, 360e, 360h, 360i, 360j, 360l, 371, 374, 381, 383). The failure to comply with any applicable provision in this part renders a device adulterated under section 501(h) of the act. Such a device, as well as any person responsible for the failure to comply, is subject to regulatory action.

Discussion

This section specifies the legal authority under which the quality system regulation requirements are written and defines the consequences for noncompliance. Failure to comply with any requirement may render the product as adulterated.

Regulatory Requirement 21 CFR § 820.1(d) Foreign Manufacturers

If a manufacturer that offers devices for import into the United States refuses to permit or allow the completion of a Food and Drug Administration (FDA) inspection of the foreign facility for the purpose of determining compliance with this part, it shall appear for purposes of section 801(a) of the act, that the methods used in, and the facilities and controls used for, the design, manufacture, packaging, labeling, storage, installation, or servicing of any devices produced at such facility that are offered for import into the United States do not conform to the requirements of section 520(f) of the act and this part and that the devices manufactured at that facility are adulterated under section 501(h) of the act.

Discussion

While the FDA does not have authority outside the United States, foreign manufacturers are required to permit or allow the FDA to inspect their facilities to ensure compliance with the quality system regulation requirements. This section states consequences foreign manufacturers will face for refusing an inspection by the FDA in that devices manufactured are adulterated under section 501(h) of the act.

Regulatory Requirement 21 CFR § 820.1 (e) Exemptions or Variances

1. Any person who wishes to petition for an exemption or variance from any device quality system requirement is subject to the requirements of section 520(f)(2) of the act. Petitions for an exemption or variance shall be submitted according to the procedures set forth in 10.30 of this chapter, the FDA's administrative procedures. Guidance is available from the Center for Devices and Radiological Health, Division of Small Manufacturers Assistance, (HFZ-220), 1350 Piccard Dr., Rockville, MD 20850, 800-638-2041 or 301-443-6597, FAX 301-443-8818.

2. The FDA may initiate and grant a variance from any device quality system requirement when the agency determines that such variance is in the best interest of the public health. Such variance will remain in effect only so long as there remains a public health need for the device and the device would not likely be made sufficiently available without the variance.

Discussion

Anyone may petition for an exemption or variance from all or part of the quality system regulation. An exemption is that a manufacturer is not required to comply, while a variance is permission to substitute a method of control different from those specified in the regulation requirements. The regulation specifies where guidance is available and how FDA priority for public health is considered.

Exemptions from GMP requirements as codified in the classification regulations 21 CFR Parts 862 to 892 will not exempt finished device manufacturers from the requirements for complaint files § 820.198 or records § 820.180.

DEFINITIONS

This section of the regulation provides definitions for terms used throughout the quality system regulation. Many of these terms will be discussed in other chapters where they are applicable to the regulation subpart.

Discussion

Section 201 of the act contains definitions considered applicable to the interpretation and implementation of the requirements in 21 CFR Part 820. For example, the terms *interstate commerce* and *device* are defined is Section 201 of the act as follows:

b. The term *interstate commerce* means: 1) commerce between any state or territory and any place outside thereof; and 2) commerce within the District of Columbia or within any other territory not organized with a legislative body.

h. The term *device* means an instrument, apparatus, implement, machine, contrivance, implant, in vitro reagent, or other similar or related article, including any component, part, or accessory that is: 1) recognized in the official National Formulary or the USP, or any supplement to them; 2) intended for use in the diagnosis of disease or other conditions, or in the cure, mitigation, treatment, or prevention of disease, in man or other animals; or 3) intended to affect the structure or any function of the body of man or other animals, and that does not achieve its primary intended purposes through chemical action within or on the body of man or other animals and that is not dependent upon being metabolized for the achievement of its primary intended purposes.

The term *component* is intended to cover all materials, including software, firmware, packaging, labeling, or assemblies, that are used as part of the finished device and are subject to component controls including; § 820.70 Receiving acceptance activities, and § 820.50 Purchasing controls.

Control number is a term commonly referred to when the manufacturer is subject to Section § 820.65 Traceability, where the device is intended for surgical implant into the body or supports or sustains life, or whose failure to perform as intended may be reasonably expected to result in serious injury. Control numbers provide linkage to the history of procurement, manufacture, packaging, labeling and distribution of units, lots, batches, or finished products. They must facilitate investigation and corrective and preventive action, including product recalls. Section § 820.184 Device History Record (DHR) applies to all devices whether § 820.65 is applicable and requires that any control number used be recorded as part of the DHR.

Establish is used throughout the regulation and requires adequate written procedures to address the requirement, and clearly states that the implementation of those procedures is also required. The definition also recognizes either electronic or paper systems, however, *Part 11 Electronic Records and Signatures* and software validation should be considered when electronic records are used.

The quality system regulation applies only to *finished devices* where the definition includes any *device* or *accessory to a device* that is suitable for use or capable of functioning. The qualifying statements "suitable for use" or "capable of functioning" differentiate a finished device from a component or assembly. For example, a manufacturer that produces a finished device intended for sale as a sterile device (capable of functioning) that has not been sterilized yet (suitable for use) is subject to the requirements as a finished device manufacturer, as is the firm that performs the sterilization.

The definition for *product* avoids repetition of other terms, such as *component, manufacturing material, finished device,* and so on throughout the regulation and is consistent with the ISO 8402:1994 definition.

The term *quality* is closely harmonized with the ISO 8402:1994 definition, adding clarity in the context of a medical device to satisfy fitness for use and safety and effectiveness.

Remanufacturers are considered manufacturers and subject to the requirements of the quality system regulation as a finished device manufacturer. Remanufacturers are those that process, condition, renovate, repackage, restore or do something to a finished device that was previously distributed, significantly changing the finished device performance or safety specifications or intended use.

The FDA adopted the ISO 8402:1994 definitions for the terms *verification* and *validation,* where verification is ensuring that outputs for a specific device or activity meet particular input requirements. Validation, a step beyond verification, includes specific intended use and requires that they are consistently fulfilled.

Specific Section Definitions

complaint—any written, electronic, or oral communication that alleges deficiencies related to the identity, quality, durability, reliability, safety, effectiveness, or performance of a device after it is released for distribution.

component—any raw material, substance, piece, part, software, firmware, labeling, or assembly that is intended to be included as part of the finished, packaged, and labeled device.

control number—any distinctive symbols, such as a distinctive combination of letters or numbers, or both, from which the history of the manufacturing, packaging, labeling, and distribution of a unit, lot, or batch of finished devices can be determined.

correction—an action taken to eliminate a detected nonconformity (for example, repair or rework). A correction can be taken in conjunction with a corrective action.

corrective action—an action taken to eliminate the cause of a detected nonconformity or other undesirable situation. Corrective action is taken to prevent recurrence of a nonconformity.

design history file (DHF)—a compilation of records that describes the design history of a finished device.

design input—the physical and performance requirements of a device that are used as a basis for device design.

design output—the results of a design effort at each design phase and at the end of the total design effort. The finished design output is the basis for the device master record. The total finished design output consists of the device, its packaging and labeling, and the device master record.

design review—a documented, comprehensive, systematic examination of a design to evaluate the adequacy of the design requirements, to evaluate the capability of the design to meet these requirements, and to identify problems.

design validation—establishing by objective evidence that device specifications conform with user needs and intended use(s).

device history record (DHR)—a compilation of records containing the production history of a finished device.

device master record (DMR)—a compilation of records containing the procedures and specifications for a finished device.

directions for use—This term provides directions under which the practitioner or layman (for example, patient or unlicensed health care provider), as appropriate, can use the device safely and for the purposes for which it is intended. Directions for use also include indications for use and appropriate contraindications, warnings, precautions, and adverse reaction information. Directions for use requirements applicable to prescription and over-the-counter devices appear throughout 21 CFR Part 801 and, in the case of in vitro diagnostic products, under 21 CFR 809.10.

establish—define, document (in writing or electronically), and implement.

finished device—any device or accessory to any device that is suitable for use or capable of functioning, whether or not it is packaged, labeled, or sterilized.

label—a display of written, printed, or graphic matter upon the immediate container of any article. [section 201(k).]

intended uses—The term "intended uses" refers to the objective intent of the persons legally responsible for the labeling of the device. The intent is determined by their expressions or may be shown by the circumstances surrounding the distribution of the device. This objective intent may, for example, be shown by labeling claims, advertising matter, or oral or written statements by such representatives. It may be shown by the offering or the using of the device, with the knowledge of such persons or their representatives, for a purpose for which it is neither labeled nor advertised. (21 CFR 801.4)

labeling—includes all labels and other written, printed, or graphic matter: 1) upon any article or any of its containers or wrappers; or 2) accompanying such article. [section 201(m).]

lot or batch—one or more components or finished devices that consist of a single type, model, class, size, composition, or software version that are manufactured under essentially the same conditions and are intended to have uniform characteristics and quality within specified limits.

management with executive responsibility—senior employees of a manufacturer who have the authority to establish or make changes to the manufacturer's quality policy and quality system.

manufacturer—any person who designs, manufactures, fabricates, assembles, or processes a finished device. Manufacturer includes, but is not limited to, those who perform the functions of contract sterilization, installation, relabeling, remanufacturing, repacking, or specification development, and initial distributors of foreign entities performing these functions.

manufacturing material—any material or substance used in or used to facilitate the manufacturing process, a concomitant constituent, or a byproduct constituent produced during the manufacturing process, which is present in or on the finished device as a residue or impurity not by design or intent of the manufacturer.

nonconformity—the nonfulfillment of a specified requirement.

preventive action—an action taken to eliminate the cause of a potential nonconformity or other undesirable potential situation. Preventive action is taken to prevent occurrence of a nonconformity.

process validation—establishing by objective evidence that a process consistently produces a result or product meeting its predetermined specifications.

product—components, manufacturing materials, in-process devices, finished devices, and returned devices.

quality—the totality of features and characteristics that bear on the ability of a device to satisfy fitness for use, including safety and performance.

quality audit—a systematic, independent examination of a manufacturer's quality system that is performed at defined intervals and at sufficient frequency to determine whether both quality system activities and the results of such activities comply with quality system procedures, that these procedures are implemented effectively, and that these procedures are suitable to achieve quality system objectives.

quality policy—the overall intentions and direction of an organization with respect to quality, as established by management with executive responsibility.

quality system—the organizational structure, responsibilities, procedures, processes, and resources for implementing quality management.

quality system record—procedures and the documentation of activities required by this part that are not specific to a particular device(s), including but not limited to the records required by § 820.20.

remanufacturer—any person who processes, conditions, renovates, repackages, restores, or does any other act to a finished device that significantly changes the finished device's performance or safety specifications, or intended use.

rework—action taken on a nonconforming product so that it will fulfill the specified DMR requirements before it is released for distribution.

specification—any requirement with which a product, process, service, or other activity must conform.

validation—confirmation by examination and provision of objective evidence that the particular requirements for a specific intended use can be consistently fulfilled.

verification—confirmation by examination and provision of objective evidence that specified requirements have been fulfilled.

where appropriate—when a requirement is qualified by "where appropriate," it is deemed to be appropriate unless the manufacturer can document justification otherwise.

MANAGEMENT RESPONSIBILITY

The requirement stated in 21 CFR § 820.5 Quality System establishes the foundation of the quality system and is stated in broad terms to allow manufacturers the flexibility necessary for implementing a quality system that is suitable and effective for their organization. The requirements in § 820.20 Management Responsibilities are the basis for responsibility, authority, and accountability over the quality system. These requirements include establishing a *quality policy*, defining the *organization structure*, appointing the *management representative*, conducting *management reviews*, *quality planning*, and *quality system procedures*.

The following section will address the individual regulatory requirement referencing the section of the quality system regulation, applicable definitions, and important points following each section.

Regulatory Requirement 21 CFR § 820.5 Quality System

Each manufacturer shall establish and maintain a quality system that is appropriate for the specific medical device(s) designed or manufactured, and that meets the requirements of this part.

Discussion

The definition for *quality system* includes not only procedures and process but also the organizational structure, responsibilities, and resources necessary to manage quality. It is also important to acknowledge the use of the term *manufacturer* and recognize that by definition, *all* finished device manufacturers are required to comply with the requirements of this part.

The requirement to define, document, and implement a quality system is consciously stated in broad terms to provide manufacturers the flexibility to design quality systems that will be appropriate and successfully implemented in their organization. What may be appropriate for one manufacturer may not be for another for the following reasons; the size of the company, the complexity of the product, the sophistication of the manufacturing process, the significance and risks associated with the product, as well as the company culture. These are factors that should be considered when designing a quality system.

Regulatory Requirement 21 CFR § 820.20 (a) Quality Policy

Management with executive responsibility shall establish its policy and objectives for, and commitment to, quality. Management with executive responsibility shall ensure that the quality policy is understood, implemented, and maintained at all levels of the organization.

Discussion

The regulation clearly places responsibility on *management with executive responsibility*, the highest-ranking member of senior management, to establish the policy and objectives for quality, ensuring the policy is understood, implemented, and maintained throughout the organization. The quality policy should reflect the overall intentions and direction of the organization with respect to quality.

Each manufacturer is different in size, culture, customers, and the product or service it provides. The quality policy should reflect the organization for which it is intended. The requirement also introduces the phrase *"objectives for quality."* Quality objectives should align with the quality policy and be stated in terms that can be measured. If quality objectives are not stated in measurable terms, it is not possible to monitor performance and commitment to achieving those objectives. The quality policy and objectives for quality are topics to be addressed at formal management reviews, where progress can be tracked and adjustments made where appropriate to ensure the policy and objectives are implemented, and maintained, as required.

The definitions, along with the requirements, make the highest accountable level of management in the organization communicate the intentions and direction for quality to all personnel. Senior management is responsible for ensuring that the quality policy is understood, implemented, and maintained at all levels of the organization. The regulation does not prescribe how to accomplish the communication of the quality policy. A variety of methods including distributing quality policy cards to all employees, all-employee communication meetings, or posting the quality policy in strategic locations throughout the facility (conference rooms, cafeterias, main reception area, and so on) will accomplish the requirement. Whichever method of communication is used, employees should be familiar with the quality policy, adhere to the direction the quality policy provides, and know where to locate it.

Regulatory Requirement 21 CFR § 820.20 (b) Organization

Each manufacturer shall establish and maintain an adequate organizational structure to ensure that devices are designed and produced in accordance with the requirements of this part.

Responsibility and authority. Each manufacturer shall establish the appropriate responsibility, authority, and interrelation of all personnel who manage, perform, and assess work affecting quality, and provide the independence and authority necessary to perform these tasks.

Resources. Each manufacturer shall provide adequate resources, including the assignment of trained personnel, for management, performance of work, and assessment activities, including internal quality audits, to meet the requirements of this part.

Management representative. Management with executive responsibility shall appoint, and document such appointment of, a member of management who, irrespective of other responsibilities, shall have established authority over and responsibility for:

(i) Ensuring that quality system requirements are effectively established and effectively maintained in accordance with this part

(ii) Reporting on the performance of the quality system to management with executive responsibility for review.

Discussion

The FDA has identified three fundamental principles essential to understanding the requirements necessary to establish and maintain an appropriate organization structure. The structure is important to ensure compliance with the quality system requirements and must also ensure the manufacturer is capable of consistently producing safe and effective devices.

1. *Responsibility and authority* requires that the organizational structure demonstrate the independence and authority of the quality function. The quality system must not be compromised as a result of the structure of the organization and reporting relationships.

2. The requirement for sufficient *resources* is broad, again recognizing the variety of finished device manufacturers that must comply with these requirements. The manufacturer is responsible for determining what is "sufficient" where all requirements of the quality system regulation are met. The term *resources* should be regarded in the broadest sense and includes personnel, supplies, sufficient funding, equipment, and so on.

3. Management with executive responsibility is responsible for documenting the appointment of the *management representative*. Documenting the appointment of the management representative does not need to be complex; it can be accomplished in a position description, quality manual, or identified on the organization chart. The responsibilities of the management representative are to ensure that the quality system is effectively implemented and to report on the performance of the quality system to management with executive responsibility. While the individual appointed to this position may have other responsibilities within the organization, it is imperative that potential conflicts that may impact the quality system are considered when this individual is selected. The responsibility and authority for the quality system must not be compromised.

Regulatory Requirement 21 CFR § 820.20(c) Management Review

Management with executive responsibility shall review the suitability and effectiveness of the quality system at defined intervals and with sufficient frequency according to established procedures to ensure that the quality system satisfies the requirements of this part and the manufacturer's established quality policy and objectives. The dates and results of quality system reviews shall be documented.

Discussion

The purpose of the management review is to provide information relevant to the overall health of the quality system, ensuring the quality policy is implemented, and that objectives for quality are being met. A written procedure is required to define how management with executive responsibility will evaluate the quality system and the frequency for such reviews. Management with executive responsibility must participate and it is expected that they act on the information, making adjustments to the quality system where necessary and providing resources to ensure its continued suitability.

The method for conducting management reviews is not specified in the regulation, allowing manufacturers the flexibility to conduct management reviews in a manner that suits their organization. Management reviews can be accomplished through a formal report, circulated to top management, or through a formal meeting. However the manufacturer chooses to conduct management reviews, the written procedure needs to describe how they are conducted and documented. The FDA will not request copies of the documented results of management reviews during a routine inspection but may request that the firm certify in writing that they have been conducted.

§ 820.100(a)(7) Corrective and Preventive Action makes a specific reference to *"Submit relevant information on identified quality problems, as well as corrective and preventive actions, for management review."* This requirement addresses decisions concerning what corrective and preventive action (CAPA) data the manufacturer will consider to be relevant for the formal management review process. The target audience should be a factor when making this decision, as the management review process is not intended to be the forum for analyzing and reviewing all CAPA data. In addition, comment 53 in the preamble identifies elements of the quality system for management review and includes the organization structure, adequacy of staffing and resources, the quality of the finished device in relation to the quality objectives, internal and external product and process performance feedback, supplier audit results, and internal audit results.

Regulatory Requirement 21 CFR § 820.20(d) Quality Planning

Each manufacturer shall establish a quality plan that defines the quality practices, resources, and activities relevant to devices that are designed and manufactured. The manufacturer shall establish how the requirements for quality will be met.

Discussion

The requirements for quality planning are specific to a product or family of products, stating how requirements for quality are met. A quality plan includes methods and resources, during all stages of manufacturing, including design, procurement, production, acceptance activities, installation, and servicing (when applicable to the manufacturer) to ensure quality requirements are met. Quality plans will tie the product's specific requirements to existing quality system procedures. They do not require the development of a new set of procedures or instructions over and above those that already exist, although the development of quality plans may identify the need for additional procedures where additional controls may be necessary.

Regulatory Requirement 21 CFR § 820.20 (e) Quality System Procedures

Each manufacturer shall establish quality system procedures and instructions. An outline of the structure of the documentation used in the quality system shall be established where appropriate.

Discussion

An outline of the structure of the documented quality system is necessary when the documentation methods are multitiered, for example, a quality manual, standard operating procedures (SOPs), or work instructions and forms. Smaller firms may have a system less complex and may satisfy the requirements with a single quality manual, quality plan, or a minimal number of written procedures. This requirement is qualified as "where appropriate" as the FDA recognizes this may not be necessary for all manufacturers. An outline should be considered appropriate when quality system documentation will require explanation to understand how related documents have been established to meet the requirements of the regulation.

DESIGN CONTROL

Design controls are defined as the systems and procedures that are incorporated into the design and development process. The use of design controls makes the design process run smoothly and clearly identifies the checkpoints and approval processes necessary to move to the next step. The use of design controls identifies discrepancies between specifications and final design results or outputs and ensures that testing processes effectively identify deficiencies in the process. Design control systems provide visibility of the design process to a company's upper management and effectively guarantee that users or customers are involved in the process of determining product specifications and ensuring that products meet those specifications.

The FDA divides the design process into the following areas:

- Design planning
- Design input
- Design output
- Design review
- Design verification
- Design validation
- Design transfer
- Design changes

PROJECT MANAGEMENT

Very few companies follow the design process precisely as described in the previous list. A typical design project does not lend itself to literal and linear following of the design control sections. More typically companies follow a design process that consists of some variation of the following sections:

- Concept

- Design and development

- Verification and validation testing

- Transfer to manufacturing

An effective design control system must integrate the regulatory requirements with the companies project development philosophy.

The following sections discuss each regulatory area, individually referencing the section of the quality system regulation and providing a list of important points following that section reference. Many of the sections that follow apply to more than one of the design process elements listed previously.

Regulatory Requirement 21 CFR § 820.30 (b) Design Input

Each manufacturer shall establish and maintain procedures to ensure that the design requirements relating to a device are appropriate and address the intended use of the device, including the needs of the user and patient.

The procedures shall include a mechanism for addressing incomplete, ambiguous, or conflicting requirements.

The design input requirements shall be documented and shall be reviewed and approved by designated individual(s).

The approval, including the date and signature of the individual(s) approving the requirements, shall be documented.

Discussion

Defining the design input or specifications for a product is the beginning of the design process. The design input forms the basis for the product design and for the methods for testing that design. Important concepts in establishing design input are:

- An effective design starts with adequate specifications.

- The more time spent clearly identifying design requirements, the less time will be spent on later design changes.

- Design input requires a combination of resources to adequately establish it—customer input, designer input, and sales and marketing input, to name a few.

Regulatory Requirement 21 CFR § 820.30(d) Design Output

Each manufacturer shall establish and maintain procedures for defining and documenting design output in terms that allow an adequate evaluation of conformance to design input requirements.

Design output procedures shall contain or make reference to acceptance criteria and shall ensure that those design outputs that are essential for the proper functioning of the device are identified.

Design output shall be documented, reviewed, and approved before release.

The approval, including the date and signature of the individual(s) approving the output, shall be documented.

Discussion

Design output is identified as the results of the design effort. It is important that the design output be expressed in terms that identify the characteristics of the design that are crucial to the safety and proper functioning of the device but are also able to be compared with design input to ensure that input requirements are met in later phases. Every document produced need not be considered part of design output, but certainly top-level documents that specify components, processes, and systems should be referenced. The following records are typically considered to be design output:

- Work products
- Block diagrams, flowcharts, software code, system or subsystem design specifications
- Product specifications
- Manufacturing procedures
- Quality assurance procedures

Regulatory Requirement 21 CFR § 820.30(e) Design Review

Each manufacturer shall establish and maintain procedures to ensure that formal documented reviews of the design results are planned and conducted at appropriate stages of the device's design development.

The procedures shall ensure that participants at each design review include representatives of all functions concerned with the design stage being reviewed and an individual(s) who does not have direct responsibility for the design stage being reviewed, as well as any specialists needed.

The results of a design review, including identification of the design, the date, and the individual(s) performing the review, shall be documented in the design history file (the DHF).

Discussion

Design reviews are intended to:

- Provide a systematic assessment of design results
- Provide feedback to designers on existing or emerging problems

- Assess project progress
- Provide confirmation that the project is ready to move on to the next stage of development
- Identify areas for further investigation and design

Review types

- Internal
- External
- Formal
- Phase related
- General design

Regulatory Requirement 21 CFR § 820.30(f) Design Verification

Each manufacturer shall establish and maintain procedures for verifying the device design. Design verification shall confirm that the design output meets the design input requirements.

The results of the design verification, including identification of the design, method(s), the date, and the individual(s) performing the verification, shall be documented in the DHF.

Discussion

Design verification and design validation are associated concepts with very important differences. Various medical device manufacturers are encouraged to use the terminology of the quality system requirements in their internal procedures. Generally, design verification is considered to be the process of verifying at each design stage that the design output conforms to defined design input requirements for that stage. Examples of this would be measuring critical dimensions of prototype components or testing the output of an electronic component. This verification process could include specific tests or evaluations and is generally performed in the laboratory or a design setting.

Regulatory Requirement 21 CFR § 820.30(g) Design Validation

Each manufacturer shall establish and maintain procedures for validating the device design. Design validation shall be performed under defined operating conditions on initial production units, lots, or batches, or their equivalents.

Design validation shall ensure that devices conform to defined user needs and intended uses and shall include testing of production units under actual or simulated use conditions.

Design validation shall include software validation and risk analysis, where appropriate.

The results of the design validation, including identification of the design, method(s), the date, and the individual(s) performing the validation, shall be documented in the DHF. Cross-reference to ISO 9001:1994 and ISO/DIS 13485 section 4.4.8 Design validation.

Discussion

While design verification has been defined as checking that design output meets design input requirements, design validation is the act of assuring that the design will conform with user needs and intended use(s). Design validation typically consists of clinical studies or simulated use of products in the laboratory. Design validation is an essential element of the design control. It requires use of the product in a setting that either simulates use or is real use (clinical studies).

Regulatory Requirement 21 CFR § 820.30(h) Design Transfer

Each manufacturer shall establish and maintain procedures to ensure that the device design is correctly translated into production specifications.

Discussion

To produce any product, a set of production specifications is used to describe the production methods for that product. Design transfer is generally considered the process of describing the production specifications that are critical to device quality documentation. The set of documentation specific to design transfer is called the device master record but could also include tests and specifications that are related to ensuring that the device as built meets the requirements for the device.

Regulatory Requirement 21 CFR § 820.30(i) Design Changes

Each manufacturer shall establish and maintain procedures for the identification, documentation, validation, or where appropriate, verification, review, and approval of design changes before their implementation.

Discussion

There can be two functional elements involved in controlling design changes:

- Document control—control of documents including tracking their status and revision history
- Change control—identification and control of changes in designs and tracking their resolution prior to design transfer

The main objectives of design changes are ensuring that:

- Corrective actions are tracked to completion.
- Changes are implemented in such a manner that the original problem is resolved.
- No new problems are created, or if new problems are created, they are also tracked to resolution.
- Design documentation is updated to accurately reflect the revised design.

Regulatory Requirement 21 CFR § 820.30(j) Design History File

Each manufacturer shall establish and maintain a DHF for each type of device.

The DHF shall contain or reference the records necessary to demonstrate that the design was developed in accordance with the approved design plan and the requirements of this part.

Discussion

There is no specific requirement in ISO 9000/1994 or ISO 13485 for a DHF. In order to market a medical device in the United States, however, a manufacturer must comply with the FDA quality system regulation, which requires a DHF.

In the previous paragraphs, a number of documents that are required have been described. The compilation of these records is the DHF.

DOCUMENTATION AND CHANGE CONTROL

Under the general requirements of this section, which state, *"Each manufacturer shall establish and maintain procedures to control all documents that are required by this part,"* manufacturers are expected to develop written procedures to describe how all product, process, and quality system documentation required by the regulation will be reviewed and approved, and subsequent changes to those documents controlled.

The requirements stated in 21 CFR § 820.40 Document Control address two basic issues:

- Document approval and distribution 21 CFR § 820.40(a)
- Document changes 21 CFR § 820.40(b)

The following section will address the individual regulatory requirement referencing the section of the quality system regulation, applicable definitions, and important points following each section.

Discussion

Throughout the regulation there are references to preparing and approving documents in accordance with the requirements of 21 CFR §' § 820.40. These references include:

- 21 CFR §' § 820.50 Purchasing Data
- 21 CFR §' § 820.70(b) Production and Process Changes
- 21 CFR §' § 820.181 Device Master Record (DMR)
- 21 CFR §' § 820.186 Quality System Record (QSR)

It is important to recognize that where the regulation makes this specific reference, the initial release of documents and any subsequent changes to those documents must be controlled under the procedures developed to meet the following requirements.

Regulatory Requirement 21 CFR § 820.40(a) Document Controls, Approval, and Distribution

Document approval and distribution. Each manufacturer shall designate an individual(s) to review for adequacy and approve prior to issuance all documents established to meet the requirements of this part. The approval, including the date and signature of the individual(s) approving the document, shall be documented. Documents established to meet the requirements of this part shall be available at all locations for which they are designated, used, or otherwise necessary, and all obsolete documents shall be promptly removed from all points of use or otherwise prevented from unintended use.

Discussion

21 CFR § 820.40(a) deals with the initial release of a document. Written procedures are required to identify an individual or group of individuals who are responsible for the review and approval of documents. The responsibilities of those individuals who review and approve documents should be clearly defined in the procedure to ensure accuracy of the document and that the document meets the requirements of the regulation. The signatures and date of the individuals approving the document must be recorded. The requirement is flexible in terms of capturing the signatures in written form or as an electronic signature, recognizing the manufacturer is obligated to meet and comply with the requirements of 21 CFR Part 11 Electronic Signatures and Records Rule.

Written procedures should describe how documents are distributed to ensure that only approved documents are available at all locations where they are used, ensuring controls are in place to either remove or otherwise prevent unintended use of superseded documents or those that have become obsolete.

Regulatory Requirement § 820.40 (b) Document Changes

Changes to documents shall be reviewed and approved by an individual(s) in the same function or organization that performed the original review and approval, unless specifically designated otherwise. Approved changes shall be communicated to the appropriate personnel in a timely manner. Each manufacturer shall maintain records of changes to documents. Change records shall include a description of the change, identification of the affected documents, the signature of the approving individual(s), the approval date, and when the change becomes effective.

Discussion

The regulation requires that individuals in the same function or organization that performed the original review and approval also review and approve changes to that document. The intent of this requirement recognizes that those individuals (same function or organization) who performed the original review and approval are typically those who possess knowledge and insight and are best suited to determine the impact the change will effect. The requirement is flexible, allowing the manufacturer the ability to specifically designate an individual(s)who did not perform the original review; however, the intent of the requirement should be achieved.

Change records are necessary not only to meet the requirements of the regulation, but also to provide the reviewers and approvers sufficient information necessary to adequately determine the impact of the change. Changes to specifications, methods, processes, or procedures specific to the product should consider, as appropriate, design verification or validation, process validation, training, regulatory submissions, as well as potential impact to distributed product. The record of change must include a description of the change being made, identify all documents affected, and the signatures and date of the approvers. The procedure must also address how the manufacturer defines "when a change becomes effective." The regulation does not prescribe how this is accomplished and leaves that decision to the manufacturer. Some manufactures use the term "effective date," which identifies the date a new document may be used. Others assign a specific lot or batch identifying when a new document may be used. Both methods will meet the requirement as long as it is described in the written procedure.

Manufacturers are responsible for implementing methods to communicate approved changes in a timely manner to ensure that affected personnel are aware of the change. Document changes are often corrections and process or product improvements that require implementation within a specified time frame. To ensure timely communication and implementation of the change, the process should recognize the significance of a change, and convey the appropriate sense of urgency based on the nature and details of the change.

PURCHASING CONTROLS

The scope of the requirements for purchasing controls include suppliers, subcontractors, and consultants, in essence all products and services that affect, directly or indirectly, the finished device or the quality system. The FDA does not regulate component suppliers and holds the finished device manufacturer accountable to ensure the products and services they purchase conform to specified requirements. The intent of the requirement is to select only those suppliers, contractors, and consultants who demonstrate the capability to provide quality products and services that meet the manufacturer's requirements and establish necessary controls to ensure the product or service conforms to specified requirements.

There are two sections to the requirements for purchasing controls. One addresses the evaluation, selection, and manufacturer controls based on the results. The second section deals with the control of purchasing data, the specified requirements for the product or service provided, and the associated purchasing documents used for procurement.

The following section will address the individual regulatory requirement referencing the section of the quality system regulation, applicable definitions, and important points following each section.

Regulatory Requirement 21 CFR § 820.50 Purchasing Controls

Each manufacturer shall establish and maintain procedures to ensure that all purchased or otherwise received product and services conform to specified requirements.

Discussion

The requirement states, "*. . . all purchased or otherwise received product and services . . .*", to understand the extent to which purchasing control requirements apply it is important to understand the definitions of *product, component,* and *manufacturing material. Product* as defined incorporates the term *component* and can include raw materials, piece parts, packaging, labels or labeling, subassemblies, and manufacturing materials. *Manufacturing materials* are those materials used during the manufacturing process but not intended to be part of the finished product. While subpart § 820.3 of the regulation does not include a definition for the term *service,* it has been discussed in the preamble under comment 102, which states *"As used in the regulation, "service" means parts of the manufacturing or quality system that are contracted to others."* Services can include: sterilization, calibration, testing, pest control, waste disposal, cleaning, environmental monitoring, installation, and so on.

Regulatory Requirement 21 CFR § 820.50 (a) Evaluation of Suppliers, Contractors, and Consultants

Each manufacturer shall establish and maintain the requirements, including quality requirements that must be met by suppliers, contractors, and consultants. Each manufacturer shall:

1. Evaluate and select potential suppliers, contractors, and consultants on the basis of their ability to meet specified requirements, including quality requirements. The evaluation shall be documented.

2. Define the type and extent of control to be exercised over the product, services, suppliers, contractors, and consultants, based on the evaluation results.

3. Establish and maintain records of acceptable suppliers, contractors, and consultants.

Discussion

The evaluation of suppliers, contractors, and consultants is presented in three basic requirements:

1. *Evaluation and selection.* Potential suppliers, contractors, and consultants must be evaluated to determine whether they are capable of meeting the manufacturer's specified requirements, including quality requirements. While the regulation does not contain a specific requirement to establish evaluation criteria, written procedures need to describe how a supplier, contractor, or consultant is evaluated and the results of the evaluation must be documented.

   The method of evaluation should be appropriate and based on the significance of the product or service in relation to the finished device. The more significant the product or service is, the more comprehensive the evaluation method should be. Methods of evaluation can include supplier audits, historical data review, or surveys.

2. *Control based on evaluation results.* Manufacturers are required to define the type and extent of control over the suppliers, contractors, and services. The level of control a manufacturer puts into practice is based on the results of the evaluation. The intent is to maintain an appropriate balance of supplier and manufacturer

controls to ensure that the product or service provided will meet requirements. For example, the manufacturer may need additional receiving acceptance controls if a supplier does not have a specific capability or is implementing corrective action as a result of nonconformity found during the evaluation process.

3. *Maintain records of acceptable suppliers.* Records of acceptable suppliers, contractors, and consultants must be maintained. The written procedure must address how records are maintained to ensure that only suppliers, contractors, and consultants who have demonstrated they are capable to meet requirements are used.

Regulatory Requirement 21 CFR § 820.50 (b) Purchasing Data

Each manufacturer shall establish and maintain data that clearly describe or reference the specified requirements, including quality requirements, for purchased or otherwise received product and services. Purchasing documents shall include, where possible, an agreement that the suppliers, contractors, and consultants agree to notify the manufacturer of changes in the product or service so that manufacturers may determine whether the changes may affect the quality of a finished device. Purchasing data shall be approved in accordance with 820.40.

Discussion

The requirement applies to the approval of purchasing data (written or electronic), including the purchasing document(s) used to procure the product or service. The specified requirements must be clear and unambiguous and approved before the data are released. Quality requirements must also be clear and unambiguous and specify the quality control and quality assurance procedures, standards, or other applicable requirements necessary to ensure the product or service is adequate for its intended use.

Purchasing documents should include, where possible, an agreement that suppliers, contractors, and consultants agree to notify the manufacturer of changes in the product or service provided. The regulation does not specify how this agreement is conveyed and can be stated on the purchase order, included in a supplier agreement, or included as part of a supplier contract. The manufacturer is ultimately responsible for the finished device and is required to review the change for potential impact on the quality of the finished device. The FDA qualifies this requirement as "where possible," recognizing that some suppliers are not willing to provide this information. However, the FDA will hold the manufacturer accountable for the quality of the finished device, and expects appropriate manufacturer controls are implemented to detect possible changes should the manufacturer consider this type of supplier acceptable.

The reference to subpart 21 CFR § 820.40 Document Control applies to all purchasing data. The DMR includes product-specific materials component specifications, manufacturing materials, packaging and labeling specifications, and so on, and is governed by the requirements of § 820.40. The specified requirements, including requirements for quality for contractors and consultants must also be controlled under the requirements of 21 CFR § 820.40.

PRODUCT IDENTIFICATION AND TRACEABILITY

Product identification and traceability requires a manufacturer to properly identify product that is manufactured and requires systems to allow traceability of the product to the manufacturing information. The specific requirements vary depending on the product type.

Regulatory Requirement 21 CFR § 820.60 Identification

Each manufacturer shall establish and maintain procedures for identifying product during all stages of receipt, production, distribution, and installation to prevent mix-ups.

Discussion

The requirement defined for identification is intentionally broad to allow the manufacturer the flexibility to use the systems for identifying its product that works best for its business. The main point is that the manufacturer provides a method to identify its materials, components, and products at all points in the process up to and including the user, and that such method(s) are formally established.

Regulatory Requirement 21 CFR § 820.65 Traceability

Each manufacturer of a device that is intended for surgical implant into the body or to support or sustain life and whose failure to perform when properly used in accordance with instructions for use provided in the labeling can be reasonably expected to result in a significant injury to the user shall establish and maintain procedures for identifying with a control number each unit, lot, or batch of finished devices and where appropriate components. The procedures shall facilitate corrective action. Such identification shall be documented in the DHR.

Discussion

The requirement for traceability applies to those devices that fall into the category of what used to be defined as "critical devices or critical components." As currently stated in the regulation, it is only required by law that any device that is "intended for surgical implant into the body or to support or sustain life and whose failure to perform when properly used in accordance with instructions for use provided in the labeling can be reasonably expected to result in a significant injury" must have a control number for each unit, lot, or batch. This requirement is not to be confused with the device tracking requirements as defined in Part 821, which require that specific medical devices be tracked to the end user by unique control number or serial number. Although traceability is only required on implants, life-supporting, or life-sustaining devices (as defined in part 820.65), it may be appropriate to apply traceability procedures to a broader population of medical devices. While it may demand the manufacturer to incur additional costs, traceability can be very beneficial when conducting a failure investigation to help isolate an incident to only those units that were affected by a certain quality problem. It is appropriate to perform a risk analysis to determine which devices are best suited to be traceable through commercialization. While the applications of this requirement have some flexibility, the manufacturer must establish procedures to assure that the approach is deployed consistently and proficiently so as to facilitate corrective action.

PRODUCTION AND PROCESS CONTROLS

Production and process controls are those techniques, procedures, and methods that are used to ensure that all processes perform as they are intended and designed. Examples of production and process controls are those procedures that document the process, any methods for monitoring processes such as statistical process control or recording of process output measurements, and workmanship standards, to name just a few. This section of the regulation also requires that production changes are controlled and that systems for calibration and control of measurement equipment are in place.

Regulatory Requirement 21 CFR § 820.70 Production and Process Controls

a. General. Each manufacturer shall develop, conduct, control, and monitor production processes to ensure that a device conforms to its specifications. Where deviations from device specifications could occur as a result of the manufacturing process, the manufacturer shall establish and maintain process control procedures that describe any process controls necessary to ensure conformance to specifications. Where process controls are needed they shall include:

1. Documented instructions, SOPs, and methods that define and control the manner of production

2. Monitoring and control of process parameters and component and device characteristics during production

3. Compliance with specified reference standards or codes

4. The approval of processes and process equipment

5. Criteria for workmanship, which shall be expressed in documented standards or by means of identified and approved representative samples

b. Production and process changes. Each manufacturer shall establish and maintain procedures for changes to a specification, method, process, or procedure. Such changes shall be verified or where appropriate validated according to Sec. 820.75, before implementation and these activities shall be documented. Changes shall be approved in accordance with Sec. 820.40.

c. Environmental control. Where environmental conditions could reasonably be expected to have an adverse effect on product quality, the manufacturer shall establish and maintain procedures to adequately control these environmental conditions. Environmental control system(s) shall be periodically inspected to verify that the system, including necessary equipment, is adequate and functioning properly. These activities shall be documented and reviewed.

d. Personnel. Each manufacturer shall establish and maintain requirements for the health, cleanliness, personal practices, and clothing of personnel if contact between such personnel and product or environment could reasonably be expected to have an adverse effect on product quality. The manufacturer shall ensure that maintenance and other personnel who are required to work temporarily under special environmental conditions are appropriately trained or supervised by a trained individual.

e. Contamination control. Each manufacturer shall establish and maintain procedures to prevent contamination of equipment or product by substances that could reasonably be expected to have an adverse effect on product quality.

f. Buildings. Buildings shall be of suitable design and contain sufficient space to perform necessary operations, prevent mix-ups, and assure orderly handling.

g. Equipment. Each manufacturer shall ensure that all equipment used in the manufacturing process meets specified requirements and is appropriately designed, constructed, placed, and installed to facilitate maintenance, adjustment, cleaning, and use.

   1. Maintenance schedule. Each manufacturer shall establish and maintain schedules for the adjustment, cleaning, and other maintenance of equipment to ensure that manufacturing specifications are met. Maintenance activities, including the date and individual(s) performing the maintenance activities, shall be documented.

   2. Inspection. Each manufacturer shall conduct periodic inspections in accordance with established procedures to ensure adherence to applicable equipment maintenance schedules. The inspections, including the date and individual(s) conducting the inspections, shall be documented.

   3. Adjustment. Each manufacturer shall ensure that any inherent limitations or allowable tolerances are visibly posted on or near equipment requiring periodic adjustments or are readily available to personnel performing these adjustments.

h. Manufacturing material. Where a manufacturing material could reasonably be expected to have an adverse effect on product quality, the manufacturer shall establish and maintain procedures for the use and removal of such manufacturing material to ensure that it is removed or limited to an amount that does not adversely affect the device's quality. The removal or reduction of such manufacturing material shall be documented.

i. Automated processes. When computers or automated data processing systems are used as part of production or the quality system, the manufacturer shall validate computer software for its intended use according to an established protocol. All software changes shall be validated before approval and issuance. These validation activities and results shall be documented.

Sec. 820.72 Inspection, measuring, and test equipment

a. Control of inspection, measuring, and test equipment. Each manufacturer shall ensure that all inspection, measuring, and test equipment, including mechanical, automated, or electronic inspection and test equipment, is suitable for its intended purposes and is capable of producing valid results. Each manufacturer shall establish and maintain procedures to ensure that equipment is routinely calibrated, inspected, checked, and maintained. The procedures shall include provisions for handling, preservation, and storage of equipment, so that its accuracy and fitness for use are maintained. These activities shall be documented.

b. Calibration. Calibration procedures shall include specific directions and limits for accuracy and precision. When accuracy and precision limits are not met, there shall be provisions for remedial action to reestablish the limits and to evaluate whether there was any adverse effect on the device's quality. These activities shall be documented.

1. Calibration standards. Calibration standards used for inspection, measuring, and test equipment shall be traceable to national or international standards. If national or international standards are not practical or available, the manufacturer shall use an independent reproducible standard. If no applicable standard exists, the manufacturer shall establish and maintain an in-house standard.

2. Calibration records. The equipment identification, calibration dates, the individual performing each calibration, and the next calibration date shall be documented. These records shall be displayed on or near each piece of equipment or shall be readily available to the personnel using such equipment and to the individuals responsible for calibrating the equipment.

Discussion

Production and process controls include all elements for producing a product that are required in order to ensure that a product meets the criteria that have been established for it during the design process. Some of the elements are fairly straightforward. For example, procedures describing how the product is to be made and the associated steps must be documented adequately. Procedure formats can vary, but the regulations require that they are reviewed and approved. The procedures could include instructions for assembly, methods for processing, inspection guidelines, or instructions. Also, a work order or other system for tracking and defining the order of the processes is needed. All manufacturing processes must be monitored. A validated process must be monitored in specific ways as described in the process validation section. However, some technique for either monitoring the result of each process on an individual component basis or periodically must be included.

All of the documentation of production processes and the processes themselves must be under change control. Any changes to the processes once they have been established must be documented and considered for either process validation or as design changes. See the appropriate section for more information.

In the event that the product can be affected by the environment, special controls must be implemented to ensure that the environment is controlled. Some products require clean rooms for reduction and control of particulate matter or control of bioburden for products to be sterilized. Any environmental controls must be documented, and validated, monitored, or verified regularly.

Buildings and associated production areas must be adequate for the purpose intended. This can take many forms, from simple assurance that product mix-ups do not take place to specific area controls for environmental reasons.

Equipment used in the manufacturing process can be classified into equipment requiring qualification as defined in the process validation section or as simpler equipment such as measuring equipment, fixtures, manufacturing aids, and so on. All equipment must be defined in a way that it can be controlled and duplicated if required. Any equipment requiring either periodic or unspecified maintenance needs a system for assuring that the maintenance is conducted as required and does not affect the quality of the product.

Personnel performing manufacturing operations must be properly trained and must be instructed on how the operation(s) being performed can affect the quality of the product. Additionally, any specific health issues must be considered.

Manufacturing operations may use material other than that specifically described in the device master record for the product. That material is typically called manufacturing material and can consist of lubricants, process aids, joining materials, and other similar products. Depending on the product type, control of manufacturing material may be required.

In the event that software is used with automated processing equipment to perform a function such as assembly or testing of the product, the software must be validated. Refer to the software section of this document for more information.

If inspection, measuring, and/or test equipment are used to manufacture product-specific controls, calibration and control of the equipment may be required. If a process can cause a deviation from the device's specification, then the process must be controlled. Additionally, processes that cannot be verified must be validated. Further discussion of process validation is in the next section. Control methods include a variety of techniques and vary from simple procedures describing the process to complex software-based systems for collecting data and providing information that can be used to adjust the process.

PROCESS VALIDATION

Process validation has long been an FDA focus and requirement. Prior to the following additions to the cGMP, the validation guidance document was the 1987 guidance intended to apply to all FDA-regulated industries. Process validation based on the 1987 guidance did not consider the "fully verified" principle that was introduced in the cGMP. The current FDA focus now follows the Global Harmonization Task Force Guidance that is much more structured toward process characterization studies and determination of process validation requirements through evaluation of the process.

Regulatory Requirement 21 CFR § 820.75 Process Validation

a. Where the results of a process cannot be fully verified by subsequent inspection and test, the process shall be validated with a high degree of assurance and approved according to established procedures. The validation activities and results, including the date and signature of the individual(s) approving the validation and where appropriate the major equipment validated, shall be documented.

b. Each manufacturer shall establish and maintain procedures for monitoring and control of process parameters for validated processes to ensure that the specified requirements continue to be met.

1. Each manufacturer shall ensure that validated processes are performed by qualified individual(s).

2. For validated processes, the monitoring and control methods and data, the date performed, and, where appropriate, the individual(s) performing the process or the major equipment used shall be documented.

c. When changes or process deviations occur, the manufacturer shall review and evaluate the process and perform revalidation where appropriate. These activities shall be documented.

Discussion

Any process validation program must begin with an evaluation of the process itself. This is best accomplished through the use of process flow diagrams or other equivalent descriptions of the process. The use of techniques, including process failure modes and effects analysis or other types of risk assessment, are also crucial to understanding the process and determining the emphasis of the process validation program.

Once the process has been described and analyzed, the next important step is to identify the verification steps in the process and any equipment and software used in the process. If the verification steps can be shown to fully verify the process (generally meaning 100 percent of the outcome of the process) then no performance qualification would be required.

Once equipment has been identified, the installation and operational qualification requirements can be established. Any major equipment (equipment that cannot be characterized solely by calibration or adjustment) must be qualified. Generally, qualification is an installation qualification ensuring that the equipment is installed correctly and operational qualification ensuring that the equipment performs the process required of it. Installation and operational qualification can be combined if it is desirable. All qualification protocols should follow a format that is predetermined and documented. All protocols should be approved in advance and executed, and then the results should be approved.

While operational qualification typically includes worst-case studies, it is not essential that worst-case studies be done. Process characterization studies to determine the operating parameters of the process precede any worst-case studies. Worst case is defined as those conditions that are within the typical operating parameters of the process. So, in general, the process characterization determines the bounds of the process and the worst-case values are those that are expected to be used in normal processing.

Following equipment qualification and the various studies, a performance qualification protocol is written and executed. The performance qualification is evidence that the process performs as designed. Therefore, all performance qualifications should take place according to procedures that will be used in normal processing. Performance qualifications must include a large enough sample to be representative of production processes.

At this point the process can be said to be qualified. However, the process has to be monitored according to the regulatory requirement, and should be in any event. Monitoring frequency can be based on the results of the various characterization and worst-case studies, and using the relative process risk determined in the process failure mode and effects analysis.

CALIBRATION

Calibration is the requirement that any equipment used for inspection, measuring, or test is suitable for its intended use. Calibration requires a means for control, procedures that describe the calibration procedures and timing, standards that are used for calibration, and records that are maintained.

Regulatory Requirement 21 CFR § 820.72 Calibration

a. Control of inspection, measuring, and test equipment. Each manufacturer shall ensure that all inspection, measuring, and test equipment, including mechanical, automated, or electronic inspection and test equipment, is suitable for its intended purposes and is capable of producing valid results. Each manufacturer shall establish and maintain procedures to ensure that equipment is routinely calibrated, inspected, checked, and maintained. The procedures shall include provisions for handling, preservation, and storage of equipment, so that its accuracy and fitness for use are maintained. These activities shall be documented.

b. Calibration. Calibration procedures shall include specific directions and limits for accuracy and precision. When accuracy and precision limits are not met, there shall be provisions for remedial action to reestablish the limits and to evaluate whether there was any adverse effect on the device's quality. These activities shall be documented.

c. Calibration standards. Calibration standards used for inspection, measuring, and test equipment shall be traceable to national or international standards. If national or international standards are not practical or available, the manufacturer shall use an independent reproducible standard. If no applicable standard exists, the manufacturer shall establish and maintain an in-house standard.

d. Calibration records. The equipment identification, calibration dates, the individual performing each calibration, and the next calibration date shall be documented. These records shall be displayed on or near each piece of equipment or shall be readily available to the personnel using such equipment and to the individuals responsible for calibrating the equipment.

Discussion

Calibration is essential to the proper manufacture of medical devices. An effective calibration program includes a system for identifying equipment requiring calibration and ensuring that recalibration takes place as required.

Calibration of equipment requires documented procedures that specify the method for calibration and the standards that are used. Standards should be traceable to a national standards organization such as the National Institute for Standards and Technology (NIST) or an equivalent. When that is not possible, an alternative is acceptable, if procedures to ensure that the alternative remains stable exist.

NONCONFORMING PRODUCT

Nonconforming product requires manufacturers to be able to identify and disposition product that has been found to be nonconforming. Disposition may vary depending on nonconformance and type of product problem.

Regulatory Requirement 21 CFR § 820.90(b) Nonconformity Review and Disposition

b. Nonconformity review and disposition

1. Each manufacturer shall establish and maintain procedures that define the responsibility for review and the authority for the disposition of nonconforming product. The procedures shall set forth the review and disposition process. Disposition of nonconforming product shall be documented. Documentation shall include the justification for use of nonconforming product and the signature of the individual(s) authorizing the use.

2. Each manufacturer shall establish and maintain procedures for rework, to include retesting and reevaluation of the nonconforming product after rework, to ensure that the product meets its current approved specifications. Rework and reevaluation activities, including a determination of any adverse effect from the rework upon the product, shall be documented in the DHR.

Discussion

Manufacturers are required to establish a procedure that provides a system for the following aspects of nonconforming product:

- Identification: this requires a means of evaluating acceptance status
- Documentation: a means to record any product that is nonconforming
- Evaluation: a review of the extent and severity of the defect
- Segregation: a place to physically store or otherwise assure restricted access
- Disposition: a cross-functional forum to make a decision on the result (that is, use as is, rework, return, or scrap of the product)

Such a process should clearly define the roles and responsibilities of the related activities, the specific requirement to investigate the root cause of the defect, and how to link this process into the corrective and preventive action system. Any investigation, as well as the disposition and corrective action, should be documented and submitted for trend analysis. It is critical that the quality data collected from this system is trended. There should then be a regular review associated with defect trends in order to prevent and correct product quality problems.

CORRECTIVE AND PREVENTIVE ACTION

According to the FDA's *Guide to Inspections of Quality Systems* (August 1999), "the purpose of the corrective and preventive action subsystem is to collect information, analyze information, identify and investigate product and quality issues, and take appropriate and effective corrective and/or preventive action to prevent their recurrence. Verifying or validating corrective and preventive actions, communicating corrective and preventive action activities to responsible people, providing relevant information for management review, and documenting these activities are essential in dealing effectively with product and quality issues, preventing their recurrence, and preventing or minimizing device failures."

Regulatory Requirement 21 CFR § 820.100 Corrective and Preventive Action

a. Each manufacturer shall establish and maintain procedures for implementing corrective and preventive action. The procedures shall include requirements for:

1. Analyzing processes, work operations, concessions, quality audit reports, quality records, service records, complaints, returned product, and other sources of quality data to identify existing and potential causes of nonconforming product, or other quality problems. Appropriate statistical methodology shall be employed where necessary to detect recurring quality problems.

2. Investigating the cause of nonconformities relating to product, processes, and the quality system.

3. Identifying the action(s) needed to correct and prevent recurrence of nonconforming product and other quality problems.

4. Verifying or validating the corrective and preventive action to ensure that such action is effective and does not adversely affect the finished device.

5. Implementing and recording changes in methods and procedures needed to correct and prevent identified quality problems.

6. Ensuring that information related to quality problems or nonconforming product is disseminated to those directly responsible for assuring the quality of such product or the prevention of such problems.

7. Submitting relevant information on identified quality problems, as well as corrective and preventive actions, for management review.

b. All activities required under this section, and their results, shall be documented.

Discussion

Section 820.100 refers to analysis of data sources to identify existing and potential causes of nonconforming product and other quality problems. A corrective and preventive action (CAPA) system is not specific to product nonconformances; it also includes process and quality system nonconformities. Manufacturers are responsible for establishing documented procedures that address all regulatory requirements for corrective and preventive action. The documented system must establish responsibility for CAPA, identify CAPA data sources, address how CAPA actions are carried out, identify how CAPA effectiveness and adequacy is verified, and allow for dissemination of information to responsible parties.

The only difference in processing a corrective action (actual) versus a preventive action (potential) is the method of identifying the data source or nonconformance. It is not necessary to have two individual systems. Corrective actions occur when an identified product or quality data source detects an actual problem. Such data sources may include:

- Acceptance activity data (component, in-process, final test)

- Product nonconformance reports

- Process performance data

- Equipment maintenance records

- Audits (internal, supplier, third party)

- Management review outputs

- Complaints

- Medical device reports

- Servicing

- Recalls

- Legal claims

Preventive actions result when analysis of the data sources (often the same as those listed previously) detect unfavorable trends. Statistical methods should be used for the analysis, as appropriate. Examples include: statistical process control charts, Pareto analysis, regression analysis, design of experiments, histograms, and scatter plots.

A CAPA program developed by medical device manufacturers must incorporate functions for handling customer complaints and returned product, servicing, post-marketing surveillance, medical device reporting, vigilance reporting, advisory notices, and removals and corrections. In addition, all quality system activities that can potentially identify a nonconformance (provide an input) need to interact with the CAPA program. Such systems include:

- Management responsibility

- Quality audit

- Design controls

- Purchasing controls

- Production and process control

- Process validation

- Acceptance activities

- Nonconforming product

- Installation

- Servicing

An effective, compliant, and "closed-loop" CAPA program will ascertain that methods are established to address the following elements.

Responsibility for Implementing the Corrective and Preventive Action System. Although CAPA procedures can delegate responsibility for the implementation and maintenance of the CAPA system to one or several functions (often quality assurance or regulatory affairs), the FDA emphasizes that it is management's responsibility to ensure that all nonconformity issues are handled appropriately. Management can show commitment to and ownership of the CAPA by providing the necessary organizational freedom for handling nonconformity issues, ensuring appropriate systems are in place, and making certain appropriate resources have been allocated.

Identification of CAPA Inputs. These inputs must include product, process, and quality data sources. Reference examples provided previously.

Documentation of CAPA Activities. Requirements for documenting the CAPA activities required by the process should be clearly spelled out in a written procedure or corresponding form. Such documentation includes: identification of the actual or potential nonconformance, a record of the investigation, the CAPA action plan, implementation and follow-up activities, and conclusions.

Analysis of Data and Investigation of the Problem. Where possible, the analysis and investigation should be taken to the level necessary to determine the root cause. A system can be established to ensure actions taken are consistent with the nonconformity type and that the degree of actions taken are proportionate to the significance of the nonconformity and the potential impacts and risks. The FDA expects procedures for assessing the risk, the actions that need to be taken for different levels of risk, and how to correct or prevent the problem from recurring, depending on that risk assessment. It is also important to note that analysis and investigation may lead to more than one solution. The rationale for choosing one solution over another should be documented.

Generation of an Action Plan. As appropriate, the CAPA action plan should consider both short- and long-term corrective and preventive actions. The action plan identifies who is responsible for implementing the action and within what time frame. When a CAPA is in response to a product nonconformity, the system must provide for control and action to be taken on suspect devices.

Implementation of the Proposed Action. The FDA expects CAPAs to be implemented in a timely fashion. An escalation process should be developed to address CAPAs that are not implemented accordingly.

Verification or Validation of Action Taken. All CAPAs require checks to ensure that actions taken were appropriate, adequate, and effective in eliminating the cause(s) of the nonconformance. These checks must also ensure that the action had no adverse effects on the product and/or system. If a CAPA is found to be inadequate or ineffective, the system should require the CAPA process to be repeated.

Communication of Action Taken. The system must allow for communication mechanisms to disseminate information to those directly responsible, including suppliers. Relevant CAPA information must also be included as an input to the management review process. Procedures should define criteria to determine what information is considered relevant for management review.

Root-Cause Investigation. In order to investigate the causes of failures, they must first be recognized. Product, process, and quality system failures and nonconformities are identifiable in several subsections of the quality system regulation, including nonconforming product (820.90), corrective and preventive action (820.100), and complaint files (820.198). All three of these quality system elements include a requirement for evaluation and investigation.

Regulatory Requirement 21 CFR § Sec. 820.90 Nonconforming Product

a. Control of nonconforming product. Each manufacturer shall establish and maintain procedures to control product that does not conform to specified requirements. The procedures shall address the identification, documentation, evaluation, segregation, and disposition of nonconforming product. The evaluation of nonconformance shall include a determination of the need for an investigation and notification of the persons or organizations responsible for the nonconformance. The evaluation and any investigation shall be documented.

21 CFR § Sec. 820.100 Corrective and preventive action

a. Each manufacturer shall establish and maintain procedures for implementing corrective and preventive action. The procedures shall include requirements for:

   2. Investigating the cause of nonconformities relating to product, processes, and the quality system

21 CFR § Sec. 820.198 Complaint files

b. Each manufacturer shall review and evaluate all complaints to determine whether an investigation is necessary. When no investigation is made, the manufacturer shall maintain a record that includes the reason no investigation was made and the name of the individual responsible for the decision not to investigate.

c. Any complaint involving the possible failure of a device, labeling, or packaging to meet any of its specifications shall be reviewed, evaluated, and investigated, unless such investigation has already been performed for a similar complaint and another investigation is not necessary.

d. Any complaint that represents an event that must be reported to FDA under part 803 or 804 of this chapter shall be promptly reviewed, evaluated, and investigated by a designated individual(s) and shall be maintained in a separate portion of the complaint files or otherwise clearly identified. In addition to the information required by Sec. 820.198(e), records of investigation under this paragraph shall include a determination of:

   1. Whether the device failed to meet specifications

   2. Whether the device was being used for treatment or diagnosis

   3. The relationship, if any, of the device to the reported incident or adverse event

e. When an investigation is made under this section, a record of the investigation shall be maintained by the formally designated unit identified in paragraph a. of this section.

Discussion

21 CFR Part 820.100 requires an analysis of the cause of nonconformities relating to product, processes, and the quality system. 820.90 requires an investigation of nonconforming product and 820.198 requires an investigation of complaints. In all cases, the activities associated with the analysis and investigation, and their results, must be documented.

Procedures for conducting failure investigation and root-cause investigation are necessary. Procedures should address the following:

Responsibilities and ownership of the process.

Systems for ensuring that the investigation is commensurate with significance and risk of the nonconformity. The extent of an investigation depends on the particular product, process, or system involved, its degree of complexity, and the risk and impact of the failure, nonconformance, or problem.

Provisions for how investigations are conducted, what records are maintained, and format requirements.

Methods for identifying the failure modes and determining the significance of the failure modes (using tools such as risk analysis).

Rationale for determining if a failure analysis should be conducted as part of an investigation. Duplicate investigations are not necessary, if it can be demonstrated that the same type of failure, problem, or nonconformity has already been investigated. In addition, the cause of failure is obvious in some cases, and a formal investigation may not be needed. If an investigation is not performed, and there is a regulatory or company requirement to do so, the reason must be documented and signed by the individual making the decision not to investigate.

Depth of the failure analysis. The depth of the analysis must be sufficient to determine the corrective action necessary to correct the problem.

An effective root-cause investigation will include the following activities:

- *Identify*—The problem, failure, or nonconformity must be clearly identified, defined, and documented.

- *Investigate*—Analyze the cause(s) of failure. All failures have a single similar property; failures adhere to the principles of cause and effect. The problem is investigated and documented, including results of the analyses, identification of the failure mode(s), and conclusions regarding root cause(s). Failure analysis should be conducted by appropriately trained and experienced personnel.

- *Act*—A thorough failure investigation should include information and other data that can be useful in developing a plan to act on the failure. Once the cause(s) have been analyzed, a firm can determine those over which one has control.

- *Document*—A record is required of the investigation, follow-up, and conclusions.

PACKAGING AND LABELING CONTROLS

One of the primary sources of recalls and problems in the medical device industry lies in the control of packaging and labeling operations. Mix-ups that occur result in product that is damaged in shipment or packaged with wrong information indicating what is in the package. These mislabeling problems can occur frequently and cause significant problems.

Regulatory Requirement 21 CFR § Sec. 820.120
Device Labeling

Each manufacturer shall establish and maintain procedures to control labeling activities.

a. Label integrity. Labels shall be printed and applied so as to remain legible and affixed during the customary conditions of processing, storage, handling, distribution, and where appropriate use:

b. Labeling inspection. Labeling shall not be released for storage or use until a designated individual(s) has examined the labeling for accuracy including, where applicable, the correct expiration date, control number, storage instructions, handling instructions, and any additional processing instructions. The release, including the date and signature of the individual(s) performing the examination, shall be documented in the DHR.

c. Labeling storage. Each manufacturer shall store labeling in a manner that provides proper identification and is designed to prevent mix-ups.

d. Labeling operations. Each manufacturer shall control labeling and packaging operations to prevent labeling mix-ups. The label and labeling used for each production unit, lot, or batch shall be documented in the DHR.

e. Control number. Where a control number is required by Sec. 820.65, that control number shall be on or shall accompany the device through distribution.

21 CFR § Sec. 820.130 Device Packaging

(a) Each manufacturer shall ensure that device packaging and shipping containers are designed and constructed to protect the device from alteration or damage during the customary conditions of processing, storage, handling, and distribution.

Discussion

These sections on labeling and packaging are very explicit. In order to have an effective system that meets the regulations, there are a number of specific requirements:

1. A procedure for approving and inspecting labeling and packaging materials by a designated individual or individuals

2. Testing of labels for integrity, generally involving ensuring that labels remain affixed

3. Control and release of stored labeling materials

4. Storage of materials to prevent mix-ups

5. Assurance that operations to label or package do not allow mix-ups

6. Assurance that any control number is properly placed

7. Validation of packaging materials to ensure that product is not damaged during shipping

These requirements can be met in a number of ways. In general, the systems for design control, incoming inspection, in-process inspection, and product manufacture must allow for labeling and packaging controls either through specific references or through general references that ensure the specific requirements have been met.

PRODUCT HANDLING, STORAGE, DISTRIBUTION, AND INSTALLATION

Product handling, storage, distribution, and installation are key areas of product manufacture, where the manufacturer must ensure that the product is handled correctly, stored correctly prior to and after distribution, and, where appropriate, installed correctly.

Regulatory Requirement 21 CFR § 820.140 Handling

Each manufacturer shall establish and maintain procedures to ensure that mix-ups, damage, deterioration, contamination, or other adverse effects to product do not occur during handling.

Regulatory Requirement 21 CFR § 820.150 Storage

a. Each manufacturer shall establish and maintain procedures for the control of storage areas and stock rooms for product to prevent mix-ups, damage, deterioration, contamination, or other adverse effects pending use or distribution and to ensure that no obsolete, rejected, or deteriorated product is used or distributed. When the quality of product deteriorates over time, it shall be stored in a manner to facilitate proper stock rotation, and its condition shall be assessed as appropriate.

b. Each manufacturer shall establish and maintain procedures that describe the methods for authorizing receipt from and dispatch to storage areas and stock rooms.

Discussion

Consideration should be given during the design phase when determining the needs of a product relative to handling and storage practices. Handling of product should be minimized relative to human contact in order to reduce any opportunity for damage, contamination, and mix-ups. Storage areas should be designed to avoid negative impact on product and maintained as such by formally established procedures. Employees who are assigned to handle product should be trained to assure that they are able to detect a quality defect and then be aware of what action to take if a defect is found. Where special environmental considerations are important for the product, those requirements must be accounted for in the design, construction, maintenance, and monitoring of the storage facilities. Similar regard should be given to the design of the containers and shelving for the product. Formally documented specifications should be established that define the storage requirements for each product. Evidence of this should be available in the quality system records for the facility.

Many times, manufacturers do not allow for handling and storage requirements beyond their own premises. It is necessary for the product to be designed to withstand all environmental conditions with which it can come into contact. Special test methods will need to have been selected and employed to assure that the product is designed, packaged, and labeled to withstand the storage and transit conditions to which it will be exposed. Where special storage and handling is required beyond the manufacturer premises, those requirements should be clearly labeled on the outside of the product container.

Regulatory Requirement 21 CFR § 820.160 Distribution

a. Each manufacturer shall establish and maintain procedures for control and distribution of finished devices to ensure that only those devices approved for release are distributed and that purchase orders are reviewed to ensure that ambiguities and errors are resolved before devices are released for distribution. Where a device's fitness for use or quality deteriorates over time, the procedures shall ensure that expired devices or devices deteriorated beyond acceptable fitness for use are not distributed.

b. Each manufacturer shall maintain distribution records that include or refer to the location of:

1. The name and address of the initial consignee

2. The identification and quantity of devices shipped

3. The date shipped

4. Any control number(s) used

Discussion

Manufacturers/distributors typically have a procedure(s) that defines the requirements of how to "pick and ship" medical devices per a customer order. Those procedures must allow for method(s) to review both the product and the customer order. The product selected should be reviewed to assure that: it matches the product number on the customer order, it is within the prescribed shelf life, the product is not damaged, and the picked quantity matches the order quantity. Where a control number is required for traceability, the procedure must also specify that requirement for the distribution record. In the event that a product is found to be nonconforming, there must be a method for handling and dispositioning the product in question. Every employee must have training records that reflect his or her ability to perform the operations as defined in those applicable procedures.

The systems employed at the point of shipment must assure that an accurate distribution record is generated for each customer. It should be possible to easily perform a product recall at the point of distribution to assure that the records are complete and accurate. It may be useful to perform a "mock" recall as part of an internal audit program. This practice would give an indication of whether, in the event of a recall, all affected products (internal and external) can be located and retrieved as quickly as possible to minimize any risk to the user and/or patient. Distribution records should be readily accessible in the event of either a quality investigation or a compliance audit. The retention, storage, and retrieval of those records should be part of the records management program for the manufacturer.

Regulatory Requirement § 820.170 Installation

a. Each manufacturer of a device requiring installation shall establish and maintain adequate installation and inspection instructions, and where appropriate, test procedures. Instructions and procedures shall include directions for ensuring proper installation so that the device will perform as intended after installation. The manufacturer shall distribute the instructions and procedures with the device or otherwise make them available to the person(s) installing the device.

b. The person installing the device shall ensure that the installation, inspection, and any required testing are performed in accordance with the manufacturer's instructions and procedures and shall document the inspection and any test results to demonstrate proper installation.

Discussion

Installation typically applies to any device that requires special instructions in order to assure that it is in working order by the manufacturer (or a contractor thereof) upon delivery. This typically means that the device requires some level of assembly or test when it arrives at a user facility. Installation should be treated no differently as a quality system requirement than any other final assembly and test procedure. Where installation applies, the manufacturer is required to assure that the installation is considered during the design of the device. This also implies a need to consider human factors not only for the use but also for the installation. The installation and associated test requirements must be formally documented as part of the DMR and provided upon delivery of the device. After the device is installed and tested those records become part of the DHR. Where an installed device fails the final test post-installation, that failure should be treated within the formal quality systems the same way any device failure is handled at final test. Any failures, investigations, reworks, and subsequent retest are also part of the DHR. Where rework must be employed, such rework procedures should be validated.

RECORDS

This section applies to all records and documents, both device-specific and quality system related, that are required by the quality system regulation. Systems are necessary to explain record management practice, identify records maintained and their location, and specify record retention periods.

There is no requirement for where records are maintained, as long as the location is known and accessible. All records must be retrievable; they should be easily located, legible, and in acceptable condition.

Regulatory Requirement 21 CFR § 820.180 General Requirements

All records required by this part shall be maintained at the manufacturing establishment or other location that is reasonably accessible to responsible officials of the manufacturer and to employees of FDA designated to perform inspections. Such records, including those not stored at the inspected establishment, shall be made readily available for review and copying by FDA employee(s). Such records shall be legible and shall be stored to minimize deterioration and to prevent loss. Those records stored in automated data processing systems shall be backed up.

a. Confidentiality. Records deemed confidential by the manufacturer may be marked to aid FDA in determining whether information may be disclosed under the public information regulation in part 20 of this chapter.

b. Record retention period. All records required by this part shall be retained for a period of time equivalent to the design and expected life of the device, but in no case less than two years from the date of release for commercial distribution by the manufacturer.

c. Exceptions. This section does not apply to the reports required by Sec. 820.20(c) Management review, Sec. 820.22 Quality audits, and supplier audit reports used to meet the requirements of Sec. 820.50(a) Evaluation of suppliers, contractors, and consultants, but does apply to procedures established under these provisions. Upon request of a designated employee of the FDA, an employee in management with executive responsibility shall certify in writing that the management reviews and quality audits required under this part, and supplier audits where applicable, have been performed and documented, the dates on which they were performed, and that any required corrective action has been undertaken.

Discussion

All records required by the quality system regulation must be stored at a location that is reasonably accessible to both the manufacturer and FDA investigators. Although records can be maintained at remote locations, the FDA expects such records to be readily available during an FDA inspection. If a foreign manufacturer maintains records at a remote site, the FDA expects those documents to be produced within a day or two.

Reproductions of required records are acceptable only if they are true and accurate copies of the original. Records may be maintained electronically, as long as the records remain protected, change controlled, and accessible. Systems are necessary to ensure electronic records are adequately backed up. Similar to other automated processes; electronic record systems must be validated.

Records may also be maintained as microfilm or microfiche reductions. Any equipment necessary for viewing and copying these records must be available.

Records deemed confidential by a manufacturer should be appropriately identified to assist the FDA in determining whether specific information may be disclosed under the Freedom of Information Act. Best practice is to only mark those records that are trade secret or proprietary information as confidential rather than routinely marking all documents provided to the FDA.

820.180(b) requires that all records, including quality records, are maintained for the life of the product, but not less than two years. This date starts upon release for commercial distribution by the manufacturer. It is up to the manufacturer to determine the shelf life and/or usable life of the device.

Meetings or reports of management review, internal quality audit reports, and supplier audit reports are not subject to FDA review. The FDA will not request to review or copy audit reports during a routine inspection. The FDA may, however, request copies of these reports in litigation under applicable procedural rules or by inspection warrant.

Regulatory Requirement 21 CFR § 820.181 Device Master Record

Each manufacturer shall maintain DMRs. Each manufacturer shall ensure that each DMR is prepared and approved in accordance with Sec. 820.40. The DMR for each type of device shall include, or refer to the location of, the following information:

a. Device specifications including appropriate drawings, composition, formulation, component specifications, and software specifications

b. Production process specifications including the appropriate equipment specifications, production methods, production procedures, and production environment specifications

c. Quality assurance procedures and specifications, including acceptance criteria and the quality assurance equipment to be used

d. Packaging and labeling specifications, including methods and processes used

e. Installation, maintenance, and servicing procedures and methods

Discussion

The DMR is intended to describe the "what" and the "how" of producing a finished device. The DMR contains the documentation for the device specifications and all other documents required for the procurement, manufacture (fabricate, assemble, mix, and so on), labeling, packaging, testing, and release of a device or family of devices. The DMR will also contain, if applicable, documents describing the sterilization, installation, and servicing of a device.

The procedures that the manufacturer places in the DMR must clearly define the requirements the manufacturer is following and when particular activities are appropriate. The DMR can be maintained as a single-source document, one or more files of the actual records, an index of these documents (noting their location), or any combination of these. Because a DMR typically contains many documents, manufacturers often use an index or bill of materials.

The contents of the DMR must be technically correct and include the most recent revisions of the documents. The DMR should also be directed toward the intended user. Evidence must exist to show that the documents have been checked for adequacy and approved for use. Changes to the DMR must be done in accordance with 820.30 and 820.40.

The listing of typical DMR documents in § 820.181 is relatively self-explanatory. Manufacturers may support the documentation by using production aids (photographs, sample assemblies, limit samples, and so on). Production aids must be identified, and be current, correct, and approved for the intended operation.

Regulatory Requirement 21 CFR § 820.184 Device History Record

Each manufacturer shall maintain DHRs. Each manufacturer shall establish and maintain procedures to ensure that DHRs for each batch, lot, or unit are maintained to demonstrate that the device is manufactured in accordance with the DMR and the requirements of this part. The DHR shall include, or refer to the location of, the following information:

a. The dates of manufacture

b. The quantity manufactured

c. The quantity released for distribution

d. The acceptance records that demonstrate the device is manufactured in accordance with the DMR

e. The primary identification label and labeling used for each production unit

f. Any device identification(s) and control number(s) used

Discussion

A DHR provides a manufacturer with traceability. The intent of the DHR is to provide evidence that the device lot or batch was manufactured in accordance with the DMR.

Although minimum requirements for a DHR are identified in § 820.184, it is not uncommon for a DHR to contain or reference the following information (as applicable to the product manufactured):

• Finished device batch, lot, control, or serial number

• Materials used and any necessary identifiers (part number, control number)

• Manufacturing dates

• Quantity started and completed

• Quantity released

• Test and inspection records

• Primary labeling

• Identification of individuals performing the operations

• Documents utilized

• References to appropriate nonconforming material reports and/or corrective and preventive actions

Unique records required for distribution under § 820.160 may also be maintained with the DHR (name and address of the initial consignee, quantity of devices shipped and date shipped).

Regulatory Requirement 21 CFR § 820.186 Quality System Record

Each manufacturer shall maintain a quality system record (QSR). The QSR shall include, or refer to the location of, procedures and the documentation of activities required by this part that are not specific to a particular type of device(s), including, but not limited to, the records required by Sec. 820.20. Each manufacturer shall ensure that the QSR is prepared and approved in accordance with Sec. 820.40.

Discussion

The QSR comprises general procedures and documentation of activities not directly related to a product or process. For many manufacturers, the QSR comprises the quality manual, lower-level SOPs, and the records documenting those activities.

COMPLAINT HANDLING

Any communication received by a manufacturer noting alleged deficiencies on a distributed product falls within the complaint handling system. The complaint handling system is not a stand-alone quality component. It is a part of a systematic approach to quality and is intricately linked with corrective and preventive action, servicing, and adverse event reporting.

Regulatory Requirement 21 CFR § 820.198 Complaint Files

(a) Each manufacturer shall maintain complaint files. Each manufacturer shall establish and maintain procedures for receiving, reviewing, and evaluating complaints by a formally designated unit. Such procedures shall ensure that:

1. All complaints are processed in a uniform and timely manner

2. Oral complaints are documented upon receipt

3. Complaints are evaluated to determine whether the complaint represents an event which is required to be reported to FDA under part 803 or 804 of this chapter, Medical Device Reporting

c. Each manufacturer shall review and evaluate all complaints to determine whether an investigation is necessary. When no investigation is made, the manufacturer shall maintain a record that includes the reason no investigation was made and the name of the individual responsible for the decision not to investigate.

d. Any complaint involving the possible failure of a device, labeling, or packaging to meet any of its specifications shall be reviewed, evaluated, and investigated, unless such investigation has already been performed for a similar complaint and another investigation is not necessary.

e. Any complaint that represents an event that must be reported to the FDA under part 803 or 804 of this chapter shall be promptly reviewed, evaluated, and investigated by a designated individual(s) and shall be maintained in a separate portion of the complaint files or otherwise clearly identified. In addition to the information required by Sec. 820.198(e), records of investigation under this paragraph shall include a determination of:

a. Whether the device failed to meet specifications

b. Whether the device was being used for treatment or diagnosis

c. The relationship, if any, of the device to the reported incident or adverse event

f. When an investigation is made under this section, a record of the investigation shall be maintained by the formally designated unit identified in paragraph (a) of this section. The record of investigation shall include:

1. The name of the device

2. The date the complaint was received

3. Any device identification(s) and control number(s) used

4. The name, address, and phone number of the complainant

5. The nature and details of the complaint

6. The dates and results of the investigation

7. Any corrective action taken

8. Any reply to the complainant

g. When the manufacturer's formally designated complaint unit is located at a site separate from the manufacturing establishment, the investigated complaint(s) and the record(s) of investigation shall be reasonably accessible to the manufacturing establishment.

h. If a manufacturer's formally designated complaint unit is located outside of the United States, records required by this section shall be reasonably accessible in the United States at either:

1. A location in the United States where the manufacturer's records are regularly kept

2. The location of the initial distributor

Discussion

In order to maintain consistency within the complaint handling process, § 820.198(a) requires that a manufacturer formally designate a complaint handling group, unit, or individual. This section also requires a manufacturer to maintain complaint files, and establish and maintain a documented procedure. The documented complaint handling procedure should address:

- Methods for receiving, reviewing, evaluating, and investigating complaints (written, electronic, or oral)

- Assignment of responsibilities for operating the system

- Corrective actions

- Maintenance of records

- Statistical analysis requirements

Manufacturers are required under § 820.198(b) to review and evaluate all complaints received to determine if the complaint is legitimate. It is during this initial review and evaluation that the manufacturer determines whether to investigate the complaint. If the decision is not to investigate, the justification must be documented.

An investigation is required if the complaint involves the alleged failure of a device (or its labeling or packaging) to meet specification *or* if the complaint meets the MDR criteria [§ 820.198(c) and (d)]. Duplicative investigations are not required if it can be shown that the same nonconformity has already been investigated. A reference to the original investigation would be considered an acceptable justification for not conducting a second investigation.

Those complaints meeting MDR reporting criteria must be clearly recognized and segregated for purposes of prioritization. Investigation records for these complaints must address the specific requirements outlined under § 820.198(d)(1) through (d)(3).

Written records of all investigations must be maintained. Complaint files and investigations should contain sufficient information to show that the report was properly reviewed and, if required, investigated. § 820.198(e) identifies the basic information that is required for all complaint investigations, including:

- Name of device

- Date complaint was received

- Reference to any control, lot, or serial numbers

- Complainant contact information

- Nature of complaint

- Results of investigation (corrective action taken, justification if no action taken, dates of investigation, name of investigator, reply, if any, to the complainant)

In most cases, manufacturers record the majority of this information [(e)(1) – (e)(5)] for all complaints received. The FDA expects manufacturers to make a "good faith" effort to obtain this data. As a result, attempted communications with the complainant to obtain missing information should be documented, whether or not the complainant responds or provides the requested information.

21 CFR § 820.198(f) requires that if the manufacturing facility is different from the formally designated complaint handling unit, the manufacturing facility receives or has access to complaint and investigation information. Firms with complaint handling units located abroad must have access to complaint files at a location within the United States [§ 820.198(g)]. In both situations, duplicate records are not required as long as there is reasonable access to the complaints and records of investigation. The manufacturer's procedures must ensure that the manufacturing site (domestic or abroad) is notified of any applicable complaints.

SERVICING

Products that can wear out in the field may require servicing and/or repair. Servicing can consist of routine maintenance or repair of defective devices.

Regulatory Requirement 21 CFR § 820.200 Servicing

a. Where servicing is a specified requirement, each manufacturer shall establish and maintain instructions and procedures for performing and verifying that the servicing meets the specified requirements.

b. Each manufacturer shall analyze service reports with appropriate statistical methodology in accordance with Section 820.100.

c. Each manufacturer who receives a service report that represents an event that must be reported to FDA under part 803 or 804 of this chapter shall automatically consider the report a complaint and shall process it in accordance with the requirements of Section 820.198.

d. Service reports shall be documented and shall include:

1. The name of the device serviced

2. Any device identification(s) and control number(s) used

3. The date of service

4. The individual(s) servicing the device

5. The service performed

6. The test and inspection data

Discussion

Servicing is typically required for reusable equipment (for example, MRI units, respirators, and wheelchairs). Where a device is defined by the manufacturer as reusable, the manufacturer is required to develop user (use, service, and maintenance) manuals as part of the finished product and as part of the DMR. Similar to the installation instructions, servicing should be considered and developed during the design phase of product development. Use and service, and maintenance instructions may be found in separate manuals, but both need to be established. Also as part of these manuals, a list of spare parts should be provided.

Service may be handled in a number of ways. Users may be qualified to perform the service and maintenance on their own, they may employ qualified staff, or they may contract this service out to a contractor or back to the original manufacturer. In any case, whenever service (preventive or corrective) is made to a medical device, there should be a documented record of that service. The records should be reviewed for statistical trends and for complaints and MDRs. Where a trend of servicing is identified that had not been previously identified and accounted for in the maintenance programs, the maintenance programs should be reviewed and upgraded as necessary.

Those service events that are not performed per planned maintenance should be considered a customer complaint. Where an incident occurs that may relate to patient hazard, an evaluation for MDR reportability should be performed and reported as required. In addition to trending and complaint review, service records are considered part of the DHR.

STATISTICAL TECHNIQUES

In typical medical device manufacturing, a variety of statistical techniques are used. Commonly a sampling plan is used for acceptance, in-process, and final inspection. That sampling plan must be based on a well-established standard and should be appropriate to the process. Statistics are used throughout the organization. Each type of statistic and the method used should be identified and documented.

Regulatory Requirement 21 CFR § 820.250 Statistical Techniques

a. Where appropriate, each manufacturer shall establish and maintain procedures for identifying valid statistical techniques required for establishing, controlling, and verifying the acceptability of process capability and product characteristics.

b. Sampling plans, when used, shall be written and based on a valid statistical rationale. Each manufacturer shall establish and maintain procedures to ensure that sampling methods are adequate for their intended use and to ensure that when changes occur the sampling plans are reviewed. These activities shall be documented.

Discussion

The requirement for statistical techniques is one of the least difficult requirements. It can be met by documenting the techniques used. However, it is more difficult to identify and use an appropriate technique. Sampling techniques have been typically based on military standards or the ANSI/ASQ Z1.4 method. But each sample chosen should have a specific basis for its choice and use. That rationale can be based on the studies done previously during process and product development. Other statistical techniques, including statistical process control and design of experiments, that are used should be developed in a similar manner.

Chapter 3

Labeling

r

LABELING REGULATION 21CFR 801

The general labeling requirements for medical devices are described in the following sections. Specific requirements for labeling, including the information to be applied to product, are contained in this section of the regulation.

Regulatory Requirement 21 CFR § 801 Labeling

The general labeling requirements for medical devices are contained in 21 CFR Part 801, Subpart A. Most recent revisions to the device labeling regulation were published in the Federal Register August 1998. This part applies only to medical devices. Subparts C, D, E, and H specify the requirements for over-the-counter devices, exemptions, and special requirements for specific devices. Those parts are not covered under the scope of this manual. In-vitro diagnostic products are addressed in 21 CFR part 809 and are also not in scope with this manual.

Regulatory Requirement: Subpart A—General Labeling Provisions 21 CFR § 801.1

Medical devices; name and place of business of manufacturer, packer or distributor.

a. The label of a device in package form shall specify conspicuously the name and place of business of the manufacturer, packer, or distributor.

b. The requirement for declaration of the name of the manufacturer, packer, or distributor shall be deemed to be satisfied, in the case of a corporation, only by the actual corporate name, which may be preceded or followed by the name of the particular division of the corporation. Abbreviations for "company," "incorporated," and so on, may be used and "the" may be omitted. In the case of an individual, partnership, or association, the name under which the business is conducted shall be used.

c. Where a device is not manufactured by the person whose name appears on the label, the name shall be qualified by a phrase that reveals the connection such person has with such device, such as, "Manufactured for _____," "Distributed by _____," or any other wording that expresses the facts.

d. The statement of the place of business shall include the street address, city, state, and zip code; however, the street address may be omitted if it is shown in a current city directory or telephone directory. The requirement for inclusion of the zip code shall apply only to consumer commodity labels developed or revised after the effective date of this section. In the case of nonconsumer packages, the zip code shall appear on either the label or the labeling (including the invoice).

e. If a person manufactures, packs, or distributes a device at a place other than his principal place of business, the label may state the principal place of business in lieu of the actual place where such device was manufactured or packed or is to be distributed, unless such statement would be misleading.

Discussion

- The label of a device shall contain the name and place of business of the manufacturer, packer, or distributor, including the street address, city, state, and zip code.

- If the firm's street address is in the local telephone directory, the street address can be omitted.

- If the firm listed on the label is not the manufacturer, the firm information must be qualified by an appropriate statement such as "Manufactured for. . . ." or "Distributed by. . . ."

Regulatory Requirement: Section 21 CFR § 801.4 Meaning of "Intended Uses"

The words "intended uses" or words of similar import in Secs. 801.5, 801.119, and 801.122 refer to the objective intent of the persons legally responsible for the labeling of devices. The intent is determined by such persons' expressions or may be shown by the circumstances surrounding the distribution of the article. This objective intent may, for example, be shown by labeling claims, advertising matter, or oral or written statements by such persons or their representatives. It may be shown by the circumstances that the article is, with the knowledge of such persons or their representatives, offered and used for a purpose for which it is neither labeled nor advertised. The intended uses of an article may change after it has been introduced into interstate commerce by its manufacturer. If, for example, a packer, distributor, or seller intends an article for different uses than those intended by the person from whom he received the devices, such packer, distributor, or seller is required to supply adequate labeling in accordance with the new intended uses. But if a manufacturer knows, or has knowledge of facts that would give him notice that a device introduced into interstate commerce by him is to be used for conditions, purposes, or uses other than the ones for which he offers it, he is required to provide adequate labeling for such a device which accords with such other uses to which the article is to be put.

Discussion

- If a packer, distributor, or seller intends a device for uses other than those intended by the person from whom he received the device, these parties must furnish adequate labeling in accordance with the new intended use.

- If a manufacturer knows or has information indicating that this device is to be used for conditions or purposes other than which it was intended, he is required to provide adequate labeling in accordance with such other uses. (An example of this might be a manufacturer of dental X-ray equipment who is routinely selling his product to podiatrists.)

Regulatory Requirement: Section 21 CFR § 801.5 Medical Devices; Adequate Directions for Use

Adequate directions for use means directions under which the layman can use a device safely and for the purposes for which it is intended. Section 801.4 defines intended use. Directions for use may be inadequate because, among other reasons, of omission, in whole or in part, or incorrect specification of:

a. Statements of all conditions, purposes, or uses for which such device is intended, including conditions, purposes, or uses for which it is prescribed, recommended, or suggested in its oral, written, printed, or graphic advertising, and conditions, purposes, or uses for which the device is commonly used; except that such statements shall not refer to conditions, uses, or purposes for which the device can be safely used only under the supervision of a practitioner licensed by law and for which it is advertised solely to such practitioner.

b. Quantity of dose, including usual quantities for each of the uses for which it is intended and usual quantities for persons of different ages and different physical conditions

c. Frequency of administration or application

d. Duration of administration or application

e. Time of administration or application, in relation to time of meals, time of onset of symptoms, or other time factors

f. Route or method of administration or application

g. Preparation for use, that is, adjustment of temperature, or other manipulation or process

Discussion

"Adequate directions for use" means directions under which the layman can use a device safely and for the purpose intended. This includes:

- Statements of all purposes for which and conditions under which the device can be used

- Quantity of dose for each use and usual quantities for persons of different ages and physical conditions

- Frequency of administration

- Duration of application

- Time of administration in relation to other factors

- Route or method of application

- Any preparation necessary for use

Regulatory Requirement: Section 21 CFR § 801.6 Medical Devices; Misleading Statements

Among representations in the labeling of a device, which render such a device misbranded, is a false or misleading representation with respect to another device, drug, food, or cosmetic.

Discussion

- A device is misbranded if it makes a false or misleading statement with respect to another device, drug, food, or cosmetic.

Regulatory Requirement: 21 CFR § 801.15 Medical Devices; Prominence of Required Label Statements

a. A word, statement, or other information required by or under authority of the act to appear on the label may lack that prominence and conspicuousness required by section 502(c) of the act by reason, among other reasons, of:

  1. The failure of such word, statement, or information to appear on the part or panel of the label that is presented or displayed under customary conditions of purchase

  2. The failure of such word, statement, or information to appear on two or more parts or panels of the label, each of which has sufficient space, and each of which is so designed as to render it likely to be, under customary conditions of purchase, the part or panel displayed

  3. The failure of the label to extend over the area of the container or package available for such extension, so as to provide sufficient label space for the prominent placing of such word, statement, or information

  4. Insufficiency of label space for the prominent placing of such word, statement, or information, resulting from the use of label space for any word, statement, design, or device that is not required by or under authority of the act to appear on the label

  5. Insufficiency of label space for the placing of such word, statement, or information, resulting from the use of label space to give materially greater conspicuousness to any other word, statement, or information, or to any design or device

6. Smallness or style of type in which such word, statement, or information appears, insufficient background contrast, obscuring designs or vignettes, or crowding with other written, printed, or graphic matter

b. No exemption depending on insufficiency of label space, as prescribed in regulations promulgated under section 502(b) of the act, shall apply if such insufficiency is caused by:

1. The use of label space for any word, statement, design, or device that is not required by or under authority of the act to appear on the label

2. The use of label space to give greater conspicuousness to any word, statement, or other information than is required by section 502(c) of the act

3. The use of label space for any representation in a foreign language

c. 1. All words, statements, and other information required by or under authority of the act to appear on the label or labeling shall appear thereon in the English language, provided, however, that in the case of articles distributed solely in the Commonwealth of Puerto Rico or in a territory where the predominant language is one other than English, the predominant language may be substituted for English.

2. If the label contains any representation in a foreign language, all words, statements, and other information required by or under authority of the act to appear on the label shall appear thereon in the foreign language.

3. If the labeling contains any representation in a foreign language, all words, statements, and other information required by or under authority of the act to appear on the label or labeling shall appear on the labeling in the foreign language.

Discussion

A word, statement, or other required information may lack the required prominence and conspicuousness for the following reasons:

- If it fails to appear on the part or panel that is displayed under customary conditions of purchase

- If the package contains sufficient space and the required information fails to appear on two or more panels, each of which is designed to render it to be displayed under customary conditions of purchase

- Failure to extend required labeling over package space provided

- Lack of sufficient label space for required labeling due to placement of nonrequired labeling of the package

- Smallness or style of type, insufficient contrast between labeling and package background, designs that obscure labeling, or overcrowding of labeling renders it unreadable

Regulatory Requirement: 21 CFR § 801.16 Medical Devices

Spanish-language version of certain required statements. If devices restricted to prescription use only are labeled solely in Spanish for distribution in the Commonwealth of Puerto Rico where Spanish is the predominant language, such labeling is authorized under Section 801.15(c).

Discussion

Where the device is restricted to prescriptions where Spanish is the prominent language, it may be generated in that language as a substitute for the English language.

Chapter 4

Medical Device Reporting

MEDICAL DEVICE REPORTING REGULATION 21CFR 803

The statutory authority for the MDR regulation is section 519 (a) of the FDCA. The final medical device reporting (MDR) regulation for user facilities was published in the *Federal Register* on December 11, 1995. On July 31, 1996, the new MDR regulation became effective for user facilities and device manufacturers. The FDA Modernization Act of 1997 (FDAMA) changes to medical device adverse event reporting became effective on February 19, 1998. On January 26, 2000, the changes to the implementing regulations, 21CFR 803 and 804, were published in the Federal Register to reflect these amendments in the act. Also, Part 804, reporting for distributors, was removed. The MDR regulation provides a mechanism for the FDA to identify and monitor significant adverse events involving medical devices, so problems may be detected and corrected in a timely manner.

The purpose of this Part 803 is to provide domestic and foreign manufacturers with:

- A thorough description of the current MDR regulation

- A clear understanding of their reporting responsibilities

- Guidance to help in the completion of the MDR forms

- An overview of required written MDR procedures, records and files

- Information on sources for forms, instructions, and other MDR information.

Scope

Under this part, device user facilities and importers must report deaths and serious injuries to which a device has or may have caused or contributed, must establish and maintain adverse event files, and must submit to the FDA specified follow-up and summary reports. Medical device distributors are also required to maintain records of such incidents.

Definitions: *Section 803.3*

a. Act means the Federal Food, Drug, and Cosmetic Act

b. Ambulatory surgical facility (ASF) means a distinct entity that operates for the primary purpose of furnishing same-day outpatient surgical services to patients. An ASF may be either an independent entity (that is, not a part of a provider of services or any other facility) or operated by another medical entity (for example, under the common ownership, licenser, or control of an entity). An ASF is subject to this regulation regardless of whether it is licensed by a federal, state, municipal, or local government or regardless of whether it is accredited by a recognized accreditation organization. If an adverse event meets the criteria for reporting, the ASF must report that event regardless of the nature or location of the medical service provided by the ASF.

c. Become aware means that an employee of the entity required to report has acquired information reasonably suggesting a reportable adverse event has occurred.

   1. Device user facilities are considered to have ``become aware'' when medical personnel, as defined in paragraph (s) of this section, who are employed by or otherwise formally affiliated with the facility, acquire such information about a reportable event.

   2. Manufacturers are considered to have become aware of an event when:

      (i) Any employee becomes aware of a reportable event that is required to be reported within 30 days or that is required to be reported within five days under a written request from the FDA under Section 803.53(b)

      (ii) Any employee, who is a person with management or supervisory responsibilities over persons with regulatory, scientific, or technical responsibilities, or a person whose duties relate to the collection and reporting of adverse events, becomes aware that a reportable MDR event or events, from any information, including any trend analysis, necessitate remedial action to prevent an unreasonable risk of substantial harm to the public health

   3. Importers are considered to have become aware of an event when any employee becomes aware of a reportable event that is required to be reported by an importer within 30 days.

d. Caused or contributed means that a death or serious injury was or may have been attributed to a medical device, or that a medical device was or may have been a factor in a death or serious injury, including events occurring as a result of: 1) failure; 2) malfunction; 3) improper or inadequate design; 4) manufacture; 5) labeling; or 6) user error.

e. 1. Device family means a group of one or more devices manufactured by or for the same manufacturer and having the same:

      (i) Basic design and performance characteristics related to device safety and effectiveness

(ii) Intended use and function

(iii) Device classification and product code

2. Devices that differ only in minor ways not related to safety or effectiveness can be considered to be in the same device family. Factors such as brand name and common name of the device and whether the devices were introduced into commercial distribution under the same 510(k) or premarket approval application (PMA), may be considered in grouping products into device families.

f. Device user facility means a hospital, ASF, nursing home, outpatient diagnostic facility, or outpatient treatment facility as defined in paragraphs (l), (b), (t), (u), and (v), respectively, of this section, which is not a "physician's office," as defined in paragraph (w) of this section. School nurse offices and employee health units are not device user facilities.

g. Distributor means, for the purposes of this part, any person (other than the manufacturer or importer) who furthers the marketing of a device from the original place of manufacture to the person who makes final delivery or sale to the ultimate user, but who does not repackage or otherwise change the container, wrapper, or labeling of the device or device package. One who repackages or otherwise changes the container, wrapper, or labeling, is a manufacturer under paragraph (o) of this section.

h. Expected life of a device (required on the manufacturer's baseline report) means the time that a device is expected to remain functional after it is placed into use. Certain implanted devices have specified "end of life" (EOL) dates. Other devices are not labeled as to their respective EOL but are expected to remain operational through maintenance, repair, upgrades, and so on, for an estimated period of time.

i. FDA means the Food and Drug Administration

j. Five-day report means an MDR that must be submitted by a manufacturer to the FDA pursuant to Section 803.53, on FDA Form 3500A or electronic equivalent as approved under Section 803.14, within five workdays.

k. Hospital means a distinct entity that operates for the primary purpose of providing diagnostic, therapeutic (medical, occupational, speech, physical, and so on), surgical and other patient services for specific and general medical conditions. Hospitals include general, chronic disease, rehabilitative, psychiatric, and other special-purpose facilities. A hospital may be either independent (for example, not a part of a provider of services or any other facility) or may be operated by another medical entity (for example, under the common ownership, licensure, or control of another entity). A hospital is covered by this regulation regardless of whether it is licensed by a federal, state, municipal, or local government or whether it is accredited by a recognized accreditation organization. If an adverse event meets the criteria for reporting, the hospital must report that event regardless of the nature or location of the medical service provided by the hospital.

l. Importer means, for the purposes of this part, any person who imports a device into the United States and who furthers the marketing of a device from the original place of manufacture to the person who makes final delivery or sale to the ultimate user, but who does not repackage or otherwise change the container, wrapper, or labeling of the device or device package. One who repackages or otherwise changes the container, wrapper, or labeling is a manufacturer under paragraph (o) of this section.

m. Malfunction means the failure of a device to meet its performance specifications or otherwise perform as intended. Performance specifications include all claims made in the labeling for the device. The intended performance of a device refers to the intended use for which the device is labeled or marketed, as defined in Section 801.4 of this chapter.

n. Manufacturer means any person who manufactures, prepares, propagates, compounds, assembles, or processes a device by chemical, physical, biological, or other procedure. The term includes any person who:

   1. Repackages or otherwise changes the container, wrapper, or labeling of a device in furtherance of the distribution of the device from the original place of manufacture

   2. Initiates specifications for devices that are manufactured by a second party for subsequent distribution by the person initiating the specifications

   3. Manufactures components or accessories that are devices that are ready to be used and are intended to be commercially distributed and intended to be used as is, or are processed by a licensed practitioner or other qualified person to meet the needs of a particular patient

   4. Is the U.S. agent of a foreign manufacturer

o. Manufacturer or importer report number means the number that uniquely identifies each individual adverse event report submitted by a manufacturer or importer. This number consists of three parts, as follows:

   1. The FDA registration number for the manufacturing site of the reported device, or the registration number for the importer. (If the manufacturing site or the importer does not have a registration number, the FDA will assign a temporary MDR reporting number until the site is officially registered. The manufacturer or importer will be informed of the temporary number.)

   2. The four-digit calendar year in which the report is submitted.

   3. The five-digit sequence number of the reports submitted during the year, starting with 00001. (For example, the complete number will appear 1234567-1995-00001.)

p. MDR means medical device report

q. MDR reportable event (or reportable event) means:

   1. An event about which user facilities become aware of information that reasonably suggests that a device has or may have caused or contributed to a death or serious injury

2. An event about which manufacturers or importers have received or become aware of information that reasonably suggests that one of their marketed devices:

    (i) May have caused or contributed to a death or serious injury

    (ii) Has malfunctioned and that the device or a similar device marketed by the manufacturer or importer would be likely to cause a death or serious injury if the malfunction were to recur

r. Medical personnel, as used in this part, means an individual who:

    1. Is licensed, registered, or certified by a state, territory, or other governing body, to administer healthcare

    2. Has received a diploma or a degree in a professional or scientific discipline

    3. Is an employee responsible for receiving medical complaints or adverse event reports

    4. Is a supervisor of such persons

t. Nursing home means an independent entity (that is, not a part of a provider of services or any other facility) or one operated by another medical entity (for example, under the common ownership, licensure, or control of an entity) that operates for the primary purpose of providing:

    (i) Skilled nursing care and related services for persons who require medical or nursing care

    (ii) Hospice care to the terminally ill

    (iii) Services for the rehabilitation of the injured, disabled, or sick

    A nursing home is subject to this regulation regardless of whether it is licensed by a federal, state, municipal, or local government or whether it is accredited by a recognized accreditation organization. If an adverse event meets the criteria for reporting, the nursing home must report that event regardless of the nature or location of the medical service provided by the nursing home.

u. 1. Outpatient diagnostic facility means a distinct entity that:

    (i) Operates for the primary purpose of conducting medical diagnostic tests on patients.

    (ii) Does not assume ongoing responsibility for patient care.

    (iii) Provides its services for use by other medical personnel. (Examples include diagnostic radiography, mammography, ultrasonography, electrocardiography, magnetic resonance imaging, computerized axial tomography and in-vitro testing.)

    2. An outpatient diagnostic facility may be either independent (that is, not a part of a provider of services or any other facility) or operated by another medical entity (for example, under the common ownership, licensure, or control of an entity).

An outpatient diagnostic facility is covered by this regulation regardless of whether it is licensed by a federal, state, municipal, or local government or whether it is accredited by a recognized accreditation organization. If an adverse event meets the criteria for reporting, the outpatient diagnostic facility must report that event regardless of the nature or location of the medical service provided by the outpatient diagnostic facility.

v. 1. Outpatient treatment facility means a distinct entity that operates for the primary purpose of providing nonsurgical therapeutic (medical, occupational, or physical) care on an outpatient basis or home healthcare setting. Outpatient treatment facilities include ambulance providers, rescue services, and home healthcare groups. Examples of services provided by outpatient treatment facilities include cardiac defibrillation, chemotherapy, radiotherapy, pain control, dialysis, speech or physical therapy, and treatment for substance abuse.

   2. An outpatient treatment facility may be either independent (that is, not a part of a provider of services or any other facility) or operated by another medical entity (for example, under the common ownership, licensure, or control of an entity). An outpatient treatment facility is covered by this regulation regardless of whether it is licensed by a federal, state, municipal, or local government or whether it is accredited by a recognized accreditation organization. If an adverse event meets the criteria for reporting, the outpatient treatment facility must report that event regardless of the nature or location of the medical service provided by the outpatient treatment facility.

w. Patient of the facility means any individual who is being diagnosed or treated and/or receiving medical care at or under the control or authority of the facility. For the purposes of this part, the definition encompasses employees of the facility or individuals affiliated with the facility, who in the course of their duties, suffer a device-related death or serious injury that has or may have been caused or contributed to by a device used at the facility.

x. Physician's office means a facility that operates as the office of a physician or other healthcare professional (for example, dentist, chiropractor, optometrist, nurse practitioner, school nurse offices, school clinics, employee health clinics, or free-standing care units) for the primary purpose of examination, evaluation, and treatment or referral of patients. A physician's office may be independent, a group practice, or part of a health maintenance organization.

z. Remedial action means, for the purposes of this subpart, any action other than routine maintenance or servicing, of a device where such action is necessary to prevent recurrence of a reportable event.

aa. 1. Serious injury means an injury or illness that:

   (i) Is life-threatening

   (ii) Results in permanent impairment of a body function or permanent damage to body structure

   (iii) Necessitates medical or surgical intervention to preclude permanent impairment of a body function or permanent damage to a body structure

2. Permanent means, for purposes of this subpart, irreversible impairment or damage to a body structure or function, excluding trivial impairment or damage.

bb. Shelf life, as required on the manufacturer's baseline report, means the maximum time a device will remain functional from the date of manufacture until it is used in patient care. Some devices have an expiration date on their labeling indicating the maximum time they can be stored before losing their ability to perform their intended function.

cc. 1. User facility report number means the number that uniquely identifies each report submitted by a user facility to manufacturers and the FDA. This number consists of three parts, as follows:

(i) The user facility's 10-digit Health Care Financing Administration (HCFA) number (if the HCFA number has fewer than 10 digits, fill the remaining spaces with zeros)

(ii) The four-digit calendar year in which the report is submitted

(iii) The four-digit sequence number of the reports submitted for the year, starting with 0001. (For example, a complete number will appear as follows: 1234560000-1995-0001.)

2. If a facility has more than one HCFA number, it must select one that will be used for all of its MDR reports. If a facility has no HCFA number, it should use all zeros in the appropriate space in its initial report (for example, 0000000000-1995-0001) and the FDA will assign a number for future use. The number assigned will be used in the FDA's record of that report and in any correspondence with the user facility. All zeros should be used subsequent to the first report if the user does not receive the FDA's assigned number before the next report is submitted. If a facility has multiple sites, the primary site can report centrally and use one reporting number for all sites if the primary site provides the name, address, and HCFA number for each respective site.

dd. Workday means Monday through Friday, excluding federal holidays

Reporting Requirements Subpart A

Regulatory Requirements: Section 803.9 Public availability of reports.

a. Any report, including any FDA record of a telephone report, submitted under this part is available for public disclosure in accordance with Part 20 of this chapter.

b. Before public disclosure of a report, FDA will delete from the report:

1. Any information that constitutes trade secret or confidential commercial or financial information under Section 20.61 of this chapter

2. Any personal, medical, and similar information (including the serial number of implanted devices), which would constitute an invasion of personal privacy under Section 20.63 of this chapter. FDA will disclose to a patient who requests a report, all the information in the report concerning that patient, as provided in Section 20.61 of this chapter

3. Any names and other identifying information of a third party voluntarily submitting an adverse event report.

c. FDA may not disclose the identity of a device user facility that makes a report under this part except in connection with:

1. An action brought to enforce section 301(q) of the act, including the failure or refusal to furnish material or information required by section 519 of the act

2. A communication to a manufacturer of a device that is the subject of a report required by a user facility under Section 803.30

3. A disclosure to employees of the Department of Health and Human Services, to the Department of Justice, or to the duly authorized committees and subcommittees of the Congress

Discussion

All reports submitted under this part are subject to public availability. Prior to any disclosure to the public, any confidential or private information will be removed with a few minor exceptions, which are also defined under this subpart.

Regulatory Requirements: Section 803.10 General Description of Reports Required from User Facilities, Importers, and Manufacturers.

a. Device user facilities. User facilities must submit the following reports, which are described more fully in subpart C of this part.

1. User facilities must submit MDR reports of individual adverse events within 10 days after the user facility becomes aware of an MDR reportable event as described in Sections. 803.30 and 803.32.

   (i) User facilities must submit reports of device-related deaths to FDA and to the manufacturer, if known.

   (ii) User facilities must submit reports of device-related serious injuries to manufacturers, or to FDA, if the manufacturer is unknown.

2. User facilities must submit annual reports as described in Section 803.33.

b. Importers must submit MDR reports of individual adverse events within 30 days after the importer becomes aware of an MDR reportable event as described in Section 803.3. Importers must submit reports of device-related deaths or serious injuries to FDA and to the manufacturer and reports of malfunctions to the manufacturer.

c. Device manufacturers. Manufacturers must submit the following reports as described more fully in subpart E of this part:

1. MDR reports of individual adverse events within 30 days after the manufacturer becomes aware of a reportable death, serious injury, or malfunction as described in Sections 803.50 and 803.52.

2. MDR reports of individual adverse events within five days of:

(i)   Becoming aware that a reportable MDR event requires remedial action to prevent an unreasonable risk of substantial harm to the public health

(ii) Becoming aware of an MDR reportable event for which FDA has made a written request, as described in Section 803.53

3. Annual baseline reports, as described in Section 803.55.

4. Supplemental reports if they obtain information that was not provided in an initial report as described in Section 803.56.

5. Annual certification to FDA of the number of MDR reports filed during the preceding year as described in Section 803.57.

Discussion

This section briefly outlines the reporting requirements for user facilities, importers, and manufacturers. There are similarities in the individual reporting and differences in the periodic reporting. Time frames vary for reporting requirements as well. Further, complete detail can be found in the subsequent sections and in the following Summary Table—Adverse Event Reporting Requirements, on page 105.

Regulatory Requirements: Section 803.11 Obtaining the Forms

User facilities and manufacturers must submit all reports of individual adverse events on FDA Form 3500A (MEDWATCH form) or in an electronic equivalent as approved under Section 803.14. This form and all other forms referenced in this section can also be obtained from the Consolidated Forms and Publications Office, Washington Commerce Center, 3222 Hubbard Rd., Landover, MD 20875; from the Food and Drug Administration, MEDWATCH (HF-2), 5600 Fishers Lane, Rockville, MD 20857, 301-827-7240; from the Division of Small Manufacturers Assistance, Office of Health and Industry Programs, Center for Devices and Radiological Health (HFZ-220), 1350 Piccard Dr. Rockville, MD 20850, FAX 301-443-8818; or fromwww.fda.gov/opacom/morechoices/fdaforms/cdrh.html.

Discussion

This section states where the forms can be obtained by reaching the agency through their address, fax number, or Web site.

Regulatory Requirements: Section 803.12 Where to Submit Reports

a. Any written report or additional information required under this part shall be submitted to: Food and Drug Administration, Center for Devices and Radiological Health, Medical Device Reporting, PO Box 3002, Rockville, MD 20847-3002.

b. Each report and its envelope shall be specifically identified, for example, "User Facility Report," "Annual Report," "Importer Report," "Manufacturer Report," "Five-Day Report," "Baseline Report," and so on.

c. If an entity is confronted with a public health emergency, this can be brought to the FDA's attention by contacting the FDA Emergency Operations Branch (HFC-162), Office of Regional Operations, at 301-443-1240, and should be followed by the submission of a fax report to 301-443-3757.

d. A voluntary telephone report may be submitted to, or information regarding voluntary reporting may be obtained from, the MEDWATCH hotline at 800-FDA-1088.

Discussion

This section states where the forms can be submitted by reaching the agency through their postal address, telephone contacts, or fax number. Electronic reporting is covered in Part 803.14.

Regulatory Requirements: 21 CFR § 803.13 English Reporting Requirement

a. All reports required in this part that are submitted in writing or electronic equivalent shall be submitted to the FDA in English.

b. All reports required in this part that are submitted on an electronic medium shall be submitted to the FDA in a manner consistent with Section 803.14.

Discussion

All reports must be submitted in writing in the English language.

Regulatory Requirements 21 CFR § 803.14 Electronic Reporting

a. Any report required by this part may be submitted electronically with prior written consent from the FDA. Such consent is revocable. Electronic report submissions include alternative reporting media (magnetic tape, disc, and so on) and computer-to-computer communication.

b. Any electronic report meeting electronic reporting standards, guidance documents, or other procedures developed by the agency for MDR reporting will be deemed to have prior approval for use.

Discussion

Electronic reporting must meet the established federal standards. Proof of this must be supplied in advance of any electronic reporting to the agency. The FDA must then give written consent prior to accepting any type of electronic reports or other communication.

Regulatory Requirements 21 CFR § 803.15 Requests for Additional Information

a. The FDA may determine that protection of the public health requires additional or clarifying information for MDRs submitted to the FDA under this part. In these instances, and in cases when the additional information is beyond the scope of FDA reporting forms or is not readily accessible, the agency will notify the reporting entity in writing of the additional information that is required.

b. Any request under this section shall state the reason or purpose for which the information is being requested, specify the date that the information is to be submitted, and clearly relate the request to a reported event. All verbal requests will be confirmed in writing by the agency.

Discussion

In the event that the FDA requires additional information beyond what was submitted on the MEDWATCH form (MDR), they should request that information in writing. The firm is responsible to either provide that additional information in the appropriate section of the MEDWATCH form 3500A or on a separate report. In either case the original MDR number must be referenced. There are many times when the original MEDWATCH form is submitted without all of the information in order to meet the established time frames. In the case where required information (as listed on the form 3500A) was not provided at the time of the original report, it is up to the firm to follow up with that information without any request from the FDA per section 803.56, Supplemental Reports.

Regulatory Requirements 21 CFR § 803.16 Disclaimers

A report or other information submitted by a reporting entity under this part, and any release by the FDA of that report or information, does not necessarily reflect a conclusion by the party submitting the report or by the FDA that the report or information constitutes an admission that the device, the reporting entity, or its employees, caused or contributed to the reportable event. The reporting entity need not admit and may deny that the report or information submitted under this part constitutes an admission that the device, the party submitting the report, or employees thereof, caused or contributed to a reportable event.

Discussion

Any report submitted under this part does not in any way constitute admission of contribution to the reportable event by the person reporting. This means that the person submitting the report does not admit guilt of committing any violation by submitting the report.

Regulatory Requirements 21 CFR § 803.17 Written MDR Procedures

User facilities, importers, and manufacturers shall develop, maintain, and implement written MDR procedures for the following:

a. Internal systems that provide for:

1. Timely and effective identification, communication, and evaluation of events that may be subject to medical device reporting requirements

2. A standardized review process/procedure for determining when an event meets the criteria for reporting under this part

3. Timely transmission of complete medical device reports to the FDA and/or manufacturers

b. Documentation and recordkeeping requirements for:

1. Information that was evaluated to determine if an event was reportable

2. All medical device reports and information submitted to the FDA and manufacturers

3. Any information that was evaluated for the purpose of preparing the submission of semiannual reports or certification

4. Systems that ensure access to information that facilitates timely follow-up and inspection by the FDA.

Discussion

User facilities, importers, and manufacturers are required to establish documented procedures to define their internal requirements for meeting the requirements of this part as it applies to their business. Additionally, files must be established and maintained at the facility to reflect that the company has met the requirements of this part. Such files must be maintained in a manner to assure they are preserved for the required time period and are readily accessible.

Regulatory Requirements: 21 CFR § 803.18 Files and Distributor Records

a. User facilities, importers, and manufacturers shall establish and maintain MDR event files. All MDR event files shall be prominently identified as such and filed to facilitate timely access.

b. 1. For purposes of this part, "MDR event files" are written or electronic files maintained by user facilities, importers, and manufacturers. MDR event files may incorporate references to other information, for example, medical records, patient files, engineering reports, and so on, in lieu of copying and maintaining duplicates in this file. MDR event files must contain:

(i) Information in the possession of the reporting entity or references to information related to the adverse event, including all documentation of the entity's deliberations and decision-making processes used to determine if a device-related death, serious injury, or malfunction was or was not reportable under this part

(ii) Copies of all MDR forms, as required by this part, and other information related to the event that was submitted to the FDA and other entities (for example, an importer, distributor, or manufacturer).

(iii) User facilities, importers, and manufacturers shall permit any authorized FDA employee during all reasonable times to access, to copy, and to verify the records required by this part.

c. User facilities shall retain an MDR event file relating to an adverse event for a period of two years from the date of the event. Manufacturers and importers shall retain an MDR event file relating to an adverse event for a period of two years from the date of the event or a period of time equivalent to the expected life of the device, whichever is greater. MDR event files must be maintained for the time periods described in this paragraph even if the device is no longer distributed.

d. 1. A device distributor shall establish and maintain device complaint records containing any incident information, including any written, electronic, or oral communication, either received by or generated by the firm, that alleges deficiencies related to the identity (for example, labeling), quality, durability, reliability, safety, effectiveness, or performance of a device. Information regarding the evaluation of the allegations, if any, shall also be maintained in the incident record. Device incident records shall be prominently identified as such and shall be filed by device, and may be maintained in written or electronic form. Files maintained in electronic form must be backed up.

   2. A device distributor shall retain copies of the records required to be maintained under this section for a period of two years from the date of inclusion of the record in the file or for a period of time equivalent to the expected life of the device, whichever is greater, even if the distributor has ceased to distribute the device that is the subject of the record.

   3. A device distributor shall maintain the device complaint files established under this section at the distributor's principal business establishment. A distributor that is also a manufacturer may maintain the file at the same location as the manufacturer maintains its complaint file under Sections. 820.180 and 820.198 of this chapter. A device distributor shall permit any authorized FDA employee, during all reasonable times, to have access to, and to copy and verify, the records required by this part.

e. The manufacturer may maintain MDR event files as part of its complaint file, under Section 820.198 of this chapter, provided that such records are prominently identified as MDR reportable events. A report submitted under this subpart A shall not be considered to comply with this part unless the event has been evaluated in accordance with the requirements of Sections. 820.162 and 820.198 of this chapter. MDR files shall contain an explanation of why any information required by this part was not submitted or could not be obtained. The results of the evaluation of each event are to be documented and maintained in the manufacturer's MDR event file.

Regulatory Requirements: Section 803.19 Exemptions, Variances, and Alternative Reporting Requirements

a. The following persons are exempt from the reporting requirements under this part:

   1. An individual who is a licensed practitioner who prescribes or administers devices intended for use in humans and who manufactures or imports devices solely for use in diagnosing and treating persons with whom the practitioner has a "physician–patient" relationship

   2. An individual who manufactures devices intended for use in humans solely for such person's use in research or teaching and not for sale, including any person

who is subject to alternative reporting requirements under the investigational device exemption regulations, parts 812 and 813 of this chapter, which require reporting of all adverse device effects

3. Dental laboratories, or optical laboratories

b. Manufacturers, importers, or user facilities may request exemptions or variances from any or all of the reporting requirements in this part. The request shall be in writing and include information necessary to identify the firm and device, a complete statement of the request for exemption, variance, or alternative reporting, and an explanation why the request is justified.

c. The FDA may grant in writing, to a manufacturer, importer, or user facility, an exemption, variance, or alternative from, or to, any or all of the reporting requirements in this part and may change the frequency of reporting to quarterly, semi-annually, annually, or other appropriate time period. These modifications may be initiated by a request as specified in this section, or at the discretion of the FDA. When granting such modifications, the FDA may impose other reporting requirements to ensure the protection of public health.

d. The FDA may revoke or modify in writing an exemption, variance, or alternative reporting requirements if the FDA determines that protection of the public health justifies the modification or a return to the requirements as stated in this part.

e. Firms granted a reporting modification by the FDA shall provide any reports or information required by that approval. The conditions of the approval will replace and supersede the reporting requirement specified in this part until such time that the FDA revokes or modifies the alternative reporting requirements in accordance with paragraph (d) of this section.

Discussion

The following persons are exempt from reporting requirements under this part:

1. An individual who is a licensed practitioner who prescribes or administers devices for human use with a specific "physician–patient" relationship

2. An individual who manufactures devices intended for use in humans solely used in research or teaching and not for sale

3. Dental or optical laboratories

Manufacturers, importers, or user facilities may submit a written request for an exemption, a variance, or alternative requirements from some or all of these requirements. The FDA may grant such request in writing; they may also revoke such exemptions, variances, or alternative requirements.

Regulatory Requirements 21 CFR § 803.20 How to Report

a. Description of form. There are two versions of the MEDWATCH form for individual reports of adverse events. FDA Form 3500 is available for use by health professionals and consumers for the submission of voluntary reports regarding FDA-regulated products. FDA Form 3500A is the mandatory reporting form to be used for submitting reports by user facilities and manufacturers of FDA-regulated products. The form has sections that must be completed by all reporters and other sections that must be completed only by the user facility, importer, or manufacturer.

1. The front of FDA Form 3500A is to be filled out by all reporters. The front of the form requests information regarding the patient, the event, the device, and the "initial reporter" (that is, the first person or entity that submitted the information to the user facility, manufacturer, or importer).

2. The back part of the form contains sections to be completed by user facilities, importers, and manufacturers. User facilities must complete section F; device manufacturers must complete sections G and H. Manufacturers are not required to recopy information submitted to them on a Form 3500A unless the information is being copied onto an electronic medium. If the manufacturer corrects or supplies information missing from the other reporter's 3500A form, it should attach a copy of that form to the manufacturer's report form. If the information from the other reporter's 3500A form is complete and correct, the manufacturer can fill in the remaining information on the same form.

b. Reporting standards

1. User facilities are required to submit MDR reports to:

    (i) The device manufacturer and to the FDA within 10 days of becoming aware of information that reasonably suggests that a device has or may have caused or contributed to a death; or

    (ii) The manufacturer within 10 days of becoming aware of information that reasonably suggests that a device has or may have caused or contributed to a serious injury. Such reports shall be submitted to the FDA if the device manufacturer is not known

2. Importers are required to submit death and serious injury reports to the FDA and the device manufacturer and submit malfunction reports to the manufacturer only:

    (i) Within 30 days of becoming aware of information that reasonably suggests that a device has or may have caused or contributed to a death or serious injury.

    (ii) Within 30 days of receiving information that a device marketed by the importer has malfunctioned and that such a device or a similar device marketed by the importer would be likely to cause or contribute to a death or serious injury if the malfunction were to recur.

3. Manufacturers are required to submit MDR reports to the FDA:

    (i) Within 30 days of becoming aware of information that reasonably suggests that a device may have caused or contributed to a death or serious injury; or

    (ii) Within 30 days of becoming aware of information that reasonably suggests a device has malfunctioned and that device or a similar device marketed by the manufacturer would be likely to cause a death or serious injury if the malfunction were to recur; or

    (iii) Within five days if required by Section 803.53.

c. Information that reasonably suggests a reportable event occurred

1. Information that reasonably suggests that a device has or may have caused or contributed to an MDR reportable event (that is, death, serious injury, and, for manufacturers, a malfunction that would be likely to cause or contribute to a death or serious injury if the malfunction were to recur) includes any information, such as professional, scientific, or medical facts and observations or opinions, that would reasonably suggest that a device has caused or may have caused or contributed to a reportable event.

2. Entities required to report under this part do not have to report adverse events for which there is information that would cause a person who is qualified to make a medical judgment (for example, a physician, nurse, risk manager, or biomedical engineer) to reach a reasonable conclusion that a device did not cause or contribute to a death or serious injury, or that a malfunction would not be likely to cause or contribute to a death or serious injury if it were to recur. Information that leads the qualified person to determine that a device-related event is or is not reportable must be contained in the MDR event files, as described in Section 803.18.

Discussion

Information that reasonably suggests that the device has or may have caused or contributed to an MDR reportable includes any information (for example, professional, scientific, or medical facts and observations or opinions) that would reasonably suggest that a device has caused or may have caused or contributed to a reportable event. MDRs are reported by medical professionals and consumers on FDA Form 3500 and by user facilities, importers, and manufacturers on FDA Form 3500A. These mandatory reporting forms have sections that must be completed by all reporters and other sections that are only required to be completed by the user facility, importer, or manufacturer.

The reporting requirements for user facilities, importers, and manufacturers are slightly different, although they are each required to use FDA forms as prescribed in Table 4.1. These reports must be submitted within the prescribed time frame either in writing or an electronic equivalent, approved by the FDA in accordance with section 803.14.

- User facilities are required to submit MDR reports to the medical device manufacturer and to submit MDR reports, as well as an annual report, to the FDA. Annual reports are submitted January 1 of each year by the user facility. These reports contain information such as HCFC provider number, user facility contact person, and specific information regarding all reportable events for that facility.

- Importers are required to submit death and serious injury reports to the FDA and malfunction reports to the manufacturer.

- Manufacturers are required to report MDR reports, baseline reports, and supplemental reports on the forms. Baseline reports are submitted when a device model is first reported under section 803.50. They contain information regarding the registration, MDR contact person, product, and market. These reports must be updated annually on the anniversary of the initial submission. Supplemental reports are used to update information on an existing MDR that was not known at the time of the initial submission of form 3500A. Foreign manufacturers must designate a U.S. agent to be responsible for reporting in accordance with section 807.40.

Table 4.1 Summary table—adverse event reporting requirements.

Reporter	What to Report	Report Form #	To Whom	When
Manufacturer/ Importer	30-day reports of deaths, serious injuries, and malfunctions	Form FDA 3500A copy to Manufacturer	FDA	Within 30 calendar days from becoming aware of an event
Manufacturer	Five-day reports on events that require remedial action to prevent an unreasonable risk of substantial harm to the public health and other types of events designated by FDA	Form FDA 3500A	FDA	Within five workdays from becoming aware of an event
Manufacturer	Baseline reports to identify and provide basic data on each device that is subject of an MDR report. At this time, FDA has stayed the requirement for denominator data requested in Part II, Items 15 and 16 on Form 3417.	Form FDA 3417	FDA	With 30 calendar, and five workday reports when device or device family is reported for the first time. Interim and annual updates are also required if any baseline information changes after initial submission.
Manufacturer	Annual certification	Form FDA 3381	FDA	Coincide with firm's annual registration dates.
User facility	Death	Form FDA 3500A	FDA & Manufacturer	Within 10 workdays
User facility	Serious injury	Form FDA 3500A	Manufacturer. FDA only if manufacturer unknown	Within 10 workdays
User facility	Annual reports of death and serious injury	Form FDA 3419	FDA	January 1

Regulatory Requirements 21 CFR § 803.21 Reporting Codes

a. The FDA has developed a MEDWATCH Mandatory Reporting Form Coding Manual for use with MDRs. This manual contains codes for hundreds of adverse events for use with FDA Form 3500A. The coding manual is available from the Division of Small Manufacturer Assistance, Center for Devices and Radiological Health, 1350 Piccard Dr., Rockville, MD 20850, fax 301-443-8818.

b. The FDA may use additional coding of information on the reporting forms or modify the existing codes on an ad hoc or generic basis. In such cases, the FDA will ensure that the new coding information is available to all reporters.

Discussion

The FDA has developed a MEDWATCH mandatory reporting form coding manual. Each MDR has a unique identifier number for tracking and trending purposes. MED-WATCH forms should be reconciled to the associated MDR so that only one MDR is filed per each event. This form coding manual is available from the Division of Small Manufacturer Assistance, CDRH.

Regulatory Requirements 21 CFR § 803.22 When Not to File

a. Only one medical device report from the user facility, importer, or manufacturer is required under this part if the reporting entity becomes aware of information from multiple sources regarding the same patient and same event.

b. An MDR that would otherwise be required under this section is not required if:

1. The user facility, importer, or manufacturer determines that the information received is erroneous in that a device-related adverse event did not occur. Documentation of such reports shall be retained in MDR files for time periods specified in Section 803.18.

2. The manufacturer or importer determines that the device was manufactured or imported by another manufacturer or importer. Any reportable event information that is erroneously sent to a manufacturer or importer shall be forwarded to the FDA, with a cover letter explaining that the device in question was not manufactured or imported by that firm.

Discussion

There are only two cases where the mandatory reporting would not be required:

1. If the reporter determines that the information they have received is erroneous (in this case it must be justified, documented, and filed in the MDR file)

2. If the reporter determines that the device was manufactured or imported by a different manufacturer or importer (in this case, the information should be forwarded to the FDA).

Regulatory Requirements: 21 CFR § 803.30 Individual Adverse Event Reports: User Facilities

a. Reporting standard. A user facility shall submit the following reports to the manufacturer or to the FDA, or both, as specified in the following:

1. Reports of death. Whenever a user facility receives or otherwise becomes aware of information, from any source, that reasonably suggests that a device has or may have caused or contributed to the death of a patient of the facility, the facility shall as soon as practicable, but not later than 10 workdays after becoming aware of the information, report the information required by Section 803.32 to the FDA, on FDA Form 3500A, or an electronic equivalent as approved under Section 803.14, and, if the identity of the manufacturer is known, to the device manufacturer.

2. Reports of serious injury. Whenever a user facility receives or otherwise becomes aware of information, from any source, that reasonably suggests that a device has or may have caused or contributed to a serious injury to a patient of the facility, the facility shall, as soon as practicable but not later than 10 workdays after becoming aware of the information, report the information required by Section 803.32, on FDA Form 3500A or electronic equivalent, as approved under Section 803.14, to the manufacturer of the device. If the identity of the manufacturer is not known, the report shall be submitted to the FDA.

b. Information that is reasonably known to user facilities. User facilities must provide all information required in this subpart C that is reasonably known to them. Such information includes information found in documents in the possession of the user facility and any information that becomes available as a result of reasonable follow-up within the facility. A user facility is not required to evaluate or investigate the event by obtaining or evaluating information that is not reasonably known to it.

Discussion

User facilities (for example, hospitals, clinics, laboratories) must report when a device has or may have caused or contributed to the death, serious illness or serious injury of a patient of the facility to the FDA and to the manufacturer (if known). They are required to submit all information known on MEDWATCH form 3500A within 10 "work" days of becoming aware of the information.

Regulatory Requirements 21 CFR § 803.32 Individual Adverse Event Reports: Data Elements

User facility reports shall contain the following information, reasonably known to them as described in 803.30(b), which corresponds to the format of FDA Form 3500A:

a. Patient information (Block A) shall contain the following:

1. Patient name or other identifier

2. Patient age at the time of event, or date of birth

    3. Patient gender

    4. Patient weight

b. Adverse event or product problem (Block B) shall contain the following:

    1. Identification of adverse event or product problem

    2. Outcomes attributed to the adverse event, for example, death, or serious injury, that is:

      (i) Life-threatening injury or illness

      (ii) Disability resulting in permanent impairment of a body function or permanent damage to a body structure

      (iii) Injury or illness that requires intervention to prevent permanent impairment of a body structure or function

    3. Date of event

    4. Date of report by the initial reporter

    5. Description of event or problem, including a discussion of how the device was involved, nature of the problem, patient follow-up or required treatment, and any environmental conditions that may have influenced the event

    6. Description of relevant tests including dates and laboratory data

    7. Description of other relevant history including preexisting medical conditions

c. Device information (Block D) shall contain the following:

    1. Brand name

    2. Type of device

    3. Manufacturer name and address

    4. Operator of the device (health professional, patient, lay user, other)

    5. Expiration date

    6. Model number, catalog number, serial number, lot number, or other identifying number

    7. Date of device implantation (month, day, year)

    8. Date of device explanation (month, day, year)

    9. Whether device was available for evaluation and whether device was returned to the manufacturer; if so, the date it was returned to the manufacturer

    10. Concomitant medical products and therapy dates. (Do not list products that were used to treat the event.)

d. Initial reporter information (Block E) shall contain the following:

    1. Name, address, and telephone number of the reporter who initially provided information to the user facility, manufacturer, or distributor

2. Whether the initial reporter is a health professional

3. Occupation

4. Whether initial reporter also sent a copy of the report to the FDA, if known

e. User facility information (Block F) shall contain the following:

1. Whether reporter is a user facility

2. User facility number

3. User facility address

4. Contact person

5. Contact person's telephone number

6. Date the user facility became aware of the event (month, day, year)

7. Type of report (initial or follow-up [if follow-up, include report number of initial report])

8. Date of the user facility report (month, day, year)

9. Approximate age of device

10. Event problem codes—patient code and device code (refer to FDA "Coding Manual for Form 3500A")

11. Whether a report was sent to the FDA and the date it was sent (month, day, year)

12. Location, where event occurred

13. Whether report was sent to the manufacturer and the date it was sent (month, day, year)

14. Manufacturer name and address; if available

Discussion

User facilities are required to complete the mandatory MEDWATCH form 3500A sections a–e as defined previously. All known information must be completed and submitted to the FDA and the manufacturer (if known) on the form within the prescribed 10-day time frame. A copy of the form should be retained at the facility.

Regulatory Requirements 21 CFR § 803.33 Annual Reports

a. Each user facility shall submit to the FDA an annual report on FDA Form 3419, or electronic equivalent as approved by the FDA under Section 803.14. Annual reports shall be submitted by January 1 of each year. The annual report and envelope shall be clearly identified and submitted to the FDA with information that includes:

1. User facility's HCFA provider number used for MDRs, or number assigned by the FDA for reporting purposes in accordance with Section 803.3(ee)

2. Reporting year

3. Facility's name and complete address

4. Total number of reports attached or summarized

5. Date of the annual report and the lowest and highest user facility report number of MDRs submitted during the report period, for example, 1234567890-1995-0001 through 1000

6. Name, position title, and complete address of the individual designated as the facility contact person responsible for reporting to the FDA and whether that person is a new contact for that facility

7. Information for each reportable event that occurred during the annual reporting period including:

   (i) User facility report number

   (ii) Name and address of the device manufacturer

   (iii) Device brand name and common name

   (iv) Product model, catalog, serial, and lot number

   (v) A brief description of the event reported to the manufacturer and/or FDA

   (vi) Where the report was submitted, that is, to the FDA, manufacturer, distributor, importer, and so on

b. In lieu of submitting the information in paragraph (a)(7) of this section, a user facility may submit a copy of FDA Form 3500A, or an electronic equivalent as approved under section 803.14, for each MDR submitted to the FDA and/or manufacturers by that facility during the reporting period.

c. If no reports are submitted to either the FDA or manufacturers during these time periods, no annual report is required.

Discussion

The FDA requires user facilities to provide an annual summary report of all MDRs on January 1 of each year for the previous year's MDRs. There is a designated FDA form 3419 that must be completed, as described previously in section 803.33, and submitted to the FDA unless there were no MDRs during that previous year.

Additional Points from the FR Notice July 23, 1996

The FDA changed the MDR requirements relative to annual certification as follows:

- The effective date of the annual certification provision of the MDR regulation for manufacturers and distributors was stayed.

- Annual certification provisions for manufacturers were stayed to allow the FDA to address industry concerns. The FDA reproposed this provision as described in the following.

- The existing requirement for distributors to annually certify was revoked (804.30). It was also reproposed, so that manufacturers and distributors would be treated the same regarding certification.

Regulatory Requirements 21 CFR § 803.40 Individual Adverse Event Reporting Requirements: Importers

Source: 65 FR 4120, Jan. 26, 2000, unless otherwise noted.

a. An importer shall submit to the FDA a report, and a copy of such report to the manufacturer, containing the information required by Section 803.42 on FDA form 3500A as soon as practicable, but not later than 30 days after the importer receives or otherwise becomes aware of information from any source, including user facilities, individuals, or medical or scientific literature, whether published or unpublished, that reasonably suggests that one of its marketed devices may have caused or contributed to a death or serious injury.

b. An importer shall submit to the manufacturer a report containing information required by Section 803.42 on FDA form 3500A, as soon as practicable, but not later than 30 days after the importer receives or otherwise becomes aware of information from any source, including user facilities, individuals, or through the importer's own research, testing, evaluation, servicing, or maintenance of one of its devices, that one of the devices marketed by the importer has malfunctioned and that such device or a similar device marketed by the importer would be likely to cause or contribute to a death or serious injury if the malfunction were to recur.

Discussion

Importers are required to report when a device has or may have caused or contributed to a death, serious illness, serious injury, or malfunction, to the FDA and to the manufacturer. They are required to submit all information known on MEDWATCH form 3500A within 30 days of becoming aware of the information.

Regulatory Requirements 21 CFR § 803.42 Individual Adverse Event Reports Data Elements

Individual medical device importer reports shall contain the information, in so far as the information is known or should be known to the importer, as described in Section 803.40, which corresponds to the format of FDA form 3500A, see also 803.32.

Discussion

Importers are required to complete the mandatory MEDWATCH form 3500A sections a–e as defined in section 803.32. All known information must be completed and submitted to the FDA and the manufacturer (if known), on the form within the prescribed 30-day time frame. A copy of the form should be retained at the facility.

Regulatory Requirements: Section 803.50 Individual Adverse Event Reports: Manufacturers.

a. Reporting standards. Device manufacturers are required to report within 30 days whenever the manufacturer receives or otherwise becomes aware of information, from any source, that reasonably suggests that a device marketed by the manufacturer:

   1. May have caused or contributed to a death or serious injury; or

   2. Has malfunctioned and such device or similar device marketed by the manufacturer would be likely to cause or contribute to a death or serious injury, if the malfunction were to recur

b. Information that is reasonably known to manufacturers.

   1. Manufacturers must provide all information required in this subpart E that is reasonably known to them. The FDA considers the following information to be reasonably known to the manufacturer:

      (i)   Any information that can be obtained by contacting a user facility, distributor, and/or other initial reporter

      (ii) Any information in a manufacturer's possession

      (iii) Any information that can be obtained by analysis, testing, or other evaluation of the device

   2. (2) Manufacturers are responsible for obtaining and providing the FDA with information that is incomplete or missing from reports submitted by user facilities, distributors, and other initial reporters. Manufacturers are also responsible for conducting an investigation of each event, and evaluating the cause of the event. If a manufacturer cannot provide complete information on an MDR report, it must provide a statement explaining why such information was incomplete and the steps taken to obtain the information. Any required information not available at the time of the report, which is obtained after the initial filing, must be provided by the manufacturer in a supplemental report under section 803.56.

Discussion

Medical device manufacturers are required to report within the prescribed 30 days any event that suggests that their device was involved in an incident that has or may have contributed to a death, serious illness, or serious injury. Additionally, manufacturers are required to report any confirmed device malfunction that, if it were to recur, would likely have a result to this effect. In any case, the manufacturer must provide all available information including the results of a failure investigation and root cause analysis. Where possible all information should be retrieved and collected from all available sources prior to the initial report of the event. Supplemental reports, providing updates of information on form 3500A, may also be forwarded to the FDA after the initial report per section 803.56.

Regulatory Requirements 21 CFR § 803.52 Individual Adverse Event Reports Data Elements

Individual medical device manufacturer reports shall contain the following information, known or reasonably known to them as described in Section 803.50(b), which corresponds to the format of FDA form 3500A, same as section 803.32 with the exception of form 3500A sections e and f as listed below.

e. All manufacturers (Block G) shall contain the following:

1. Contact office name and address and device manufacturing site

2. Telephone number

3. Report sources

4. Date received by manufacturer (month, day, year)

5. Type of report being submitted (for example, five-day, initial, supplemental)

6. Manufacturer report number

f. Device manufacturers (Block H) shall contain the following:

1. Type of reportable event (death, serious injury, malfunction, and so on)

2. Type of follow-up report, if applicable (for example, correction, response to FDA request, and so on)

3. If the device was returned to the manufacturer and evaluated by the manufacturer, a summary of the evaluation. If no evaluation was performed, provide an explanation why no evaluation was performed

4. Device manufacture date (month, day, year)

5. Was device labeled for single use

6. Evaluation codes (including event codes, method of evaluation, result, and conclusion codes) (refer to FDA "Coding Manual for Form 3500A")

7. Whether remedial action was taken and type

8. Whether use of device was initial, reuse, or unknown

9. Whether remedial action was reported as a removal or correction under section 519(f) of the act (list the correction/removal report number)

10. Additional manufacturer narrative; and/or (11) corrected data, including:

    (i) Any information missing on the user facility report or distributor report, including missing event codes, or information corrected on such forms after manufacturer verification

    (ii) For each event code provided by the user facility under Section 803.32(d)(10) or a distributor, a statement of whether the type of the event represented by the code is addressed in the device labeling

    (iii) If any required information was not provided, an explanation of why such information was not provided and the steps taken to obtain such information

Discussion

Manufacturers are required to complete the mandatory MEDWATCH form 3500A sections a–e as defined in section 803.32 as well as f–g in section 803.52. All known information must be completed and submitted to the FDA, on the form within the 30-day allowed time frame. The exception to this is where either the information necessitates remedial action to prevent an unreasonable risk of substantial harm to the public health or in a case where the FDA has made a written request for the submission of a five-day report. A copy of the form must be retained at the facility.

Regulatory Requirements: Section 803.53 Five-Day Reports

A manufacturer shall submit a five-day report to the FDA, on form 3500A or electronic equivalent as approved by the FDA under Section 803.14 within five workdays of:

a. Becoming aware that a reportable MDR event or events, from any information, including any trend analysis, necessitates remedial action to prevent an unreasonable risk of substantial harm to the public health; or

b. Becoming aware of an MDR reportable event for which the FDA has made a written request for the submission of a five-day report. When such a request is made, the manufacturer shall submit, without further requests, a five-day report for all subsequent events of the same nature that involve substantially similar devices for the time period specified in the written request. The time period stated in the original written request can be extended by the FDA if it is in the interest of the public health.

Discussion

Manufacturers are required to submit a five-day report when either the information necessitates remedial action to prevent an unreasonable risk of substantial harm to the public health or in a case where the FDA has made a written request for the submission of a five-day report. The report should be submitted on the form 3500A. A copy of the form must be retained at the facility.

Regulatory Requirements 21 CFR § 803.55 Baseline Reports

a. A manufacturer shall submit a baseline report on FDA form 3417, or electronic equivalent as approved by the FDA under Section 803.14 for a device when the device model is first reported under Section 803.50.

b. Each baseline report shall be updated annually, on the anniversary month of the initial submission, after the initial baseline report is submitted. Changes to baseline information shall be reported in the manner described in Section 803.56 (that is, include only the new, changed, or corrected information in the appropriate portion(s) of the report form). Baseline reports shall contain the following:

    1. Name, complete address, and registration number of the manufacturer's reporting site. If the reporting site is not registered, the FDA will assign a temporary registration number until the reporting site officially registers. The manufacturer will be informed of the temporary registration number

2. FDA registration number of each site where the device is manufactured

3. Name, complete address, and telephone number of the individual who has been designated by the manufacturer as its MDR contact and date of the report. For foreign manufacturers, a confirmation that the individual submitting the report is the agent of the manufacturer designated under Section 803.58(a) is required.

4. Product identification, including device family, brand name, generic name, model number, catalog number, product code, and any other product identification number or designation

5. Identification of any device previously reported in a baseline report that is substantially similar (for example, same device with a different model number, or same device except for cosmetic differences in color or shape) to the device being reported, including the identification of the previously reported device by model number, catalog number, or other product identification, and the date of the baseline report for the previously reported device

6. Basis for marketing, including 510(k) premarket notification number or PMA number, if applicable, and whether the device is currently the subject of an approved post-market study under section 522 of the act

7. Date the device was initially marketed and, if applicable, the date on which the manufacturer ceased marketing the device

8. Shelf life, if applicable, and expected life of the device

9. The number of devices manufactured and distributed in the last 12 months and, an estimate of the number of devices in current use

10. Brief description of any methods used to estimate the number of devices distributed and the method used to estimate the number of devices in current use. If this information was provided in a previous baseline report, in lieu of resubmitting the information, it may be referenced by providing the date and product identification for the previous baseline report

Discussion

A baseline report must be submitted to the FDA for each product family upon the first MDR reportable event. The specific required information is outlined on FDA form 3417. This report should be updated once annually on the anniversary of the first report with any new or changed information for that product.

Additional Points As Published in the FR Notice on July 31, 1996

The FDA placed into abeyance, or stayed, the effective date of the provision of the MDR regulation that relates to part of the baseline reporting requirement [21 CFR 803.55(b)(9) and (10)]. Therefore, at this time, the FDA will not require any manufacturer to submit denominator data requested in Part II, Items 15 and 16 only on form FDA 3417, "Baseline Report." Instead, the FDA will initiate a demonstration project to evaluate denominator data. At the completion of this project, the FDA will lift the stay, retain it, or repropose these specific requirements.

Regulatory Reports 21 CFR § 803.56 Supplemental Reports

When a manufacturer obtains information required under this part that was not provided because it was not known or was not available when the initial report was submitted, the manufacturer shall submit to the FDA the supplemental information within one month following receipt of such information. In supplemental reports, the manufacturer shall:

a. Indicate on the form and the envelope, that the reporting form being submitted is a supplemental report. If the report being supplemented is an FDA form 3500A report, the manufacturer must select, in Item H-2, the appropriate code for the type of supplemental information being submitted

b. Provide the appropriate identification numbers of the report that will be updated with the supplemental information, for example, original manufacturer report number and user facility report number, if applicable

c. For reports that cross-reference previous reports, include only the new, changed, or corrected information in the appropriate portion(s) of the respective form(s).

Discussion

Any information that was not provided in the original MDR (MEDWATCH form) must be submitted to the FDA with reference to the original MDR number within one month of becoming aware of the information. The supplemental information must be provided in the specific format indicated previously. In order to be clear and efficient, it is important to only provide the new or changed information, with reference to the original report (MEDWATCH form) number and clearly refer to the fact that it is a supplemental report on both the report and the outer envelope.

Regulatory Requirements: 21 CFR § 803.58 Foreign Manufacturers

a. Every foreign manufacturer whose devices are distributed in the United States shall designate a U.S. agent to be responsible for reporting in accordance with Section 807.40 of this chapter. The U.S.-designated agent accepts responsibility for the duties that such designation entails. Upon the effective date of this regulation, foreign manufacturers shall inform the FDA, by letter, of the name and address of the U.S. agent designated under this section and Section 807.40 of this chapter, and shall update this information as necessary. Such updated information shall be submitted to the FDA, within five days of a change in the designated agent information.

b. U.S.-designated agents of foreign manufacturers are required to:

1. Report to the FDA in accordance with Sections. 803.50, 803.52, 803.53, 803.55, and 803.56

2. Conduct or obtain from the foreign manufacturer the necessary information regarding the investigation and evaluation of the event to comport with the requirements of Section 803.50

3. Certify in accordance with Section 803.57

4. Forward MDR complaints to the foreign manufacturer and maintain documentation of this requirement

5. Maintain complaint files in accordance with Section 803.18

6. Register, list, and submit premarket notifications in accordance with part 807 of this chapter

Discussion

The FDA began to receive comments regarding the regulation, following publication of the December 11, 1995, final rule on MDR for manufacturers and user facilities. The FDA staff subsequently met with industry representatives to discuss their concerns about the new regulation. Following these discussions, the FDA decided to place all or portions of three specific parts of the regulation into abeyance. This means that the FDA has revoked/stayed, or delayed these parts from going into effect.

Therefore:

1. Foreign manufacturers are not required to have a U.S.-designated agent (USDA).

2. There is no requirement to submit distribution information dictated by sections 803.55(b)(9) and (10) of the baseline reporting requirement. This means that manufacturers do not fill out data elements 15 and 16 only of the baseline report (form FDA 3417).

3. A foreign manufacturer is fully subject to the MDR requirements. If a foreign manufacturer already has a USDA, it may forward MDRs through this agent until further notice. However, if a foreign manufacturer chooses to employ a contact in the United States to forward reports to the FDA, the FDA views this person as if he or she is an employee of the foreign firm. The FDA explains these decisions in the *Federal Register (FR)* notices summarized below.

4. The FDA encourages foreign firms to register with the FDA by completing a form FDA 2891, "Initial Registration of Device Establishment."

Additional Points from the Modernization Act Changes, Effective February 19, 1998

- *Distributors.* Distributors of medical devices are no longer required to report device-related adverse events involving death, serious injury, and malfunction to the FDA and/or the device manufacturer. Instead, distributors must keep records of complaints and make the records available to the FDA upon request.

- *Annual certification requirement.* The annual certification requirement repeals the requirement for manufacturers, importers, and distributors to submit an annual certification, form FDA 3381, to the FDA certifying whether any adverse event reports were filed during the previous year and, if so, the number filed.

- *User facilities.* The user facility semi-annual reporting requirement has been changed to annual reporting. The annual report will now be due on January 1 of each year. User facilities may continue to use the current semiannual user facility report form, FDA 3419, until a revised one is issued by the FDA.

The identity of user facilities that are submitting MDR reports is protected from disclosure except in connection with:

1. Certain actions brought to enforce device requirements under the FFD&C Act

2. A communication to a manufacturer of a device that is the subject of a report to the FDA of death, serious illness or injury, or other significant adverse experience

Chapter 5
Recalls, Corrections, and Removals

R ecalls are a method for companies to remove product from the market in cases where the product has been shown to not meet its specified requirements. Recalls can consist of notification to users or actual removal of product. The FDA has specific requirements for recalls that are described in the following sections.

VOLUNTARY RECALLS

A voluntary recall is an alternative to waiting for the FDA to order one. There are several clear benefits, including:

- The manufacturer controls the method of the recall

- Generally, they are more efficient

- Most people want to fix what's wrong

- Many more want to stay on good terms with the FDA

- Most people want to avoid lawsuits

If the recall is successful there is one mention in the FDA enforcement report.

One of the better voluntary recalls and one that serves as a model is Johnson & Johnson's experience with Tylenol.

Position of the FDA

There are several incentives for a company to recall a product, including the moral duty to protect its customers from harm and the desire to avoid private lawsuits if injuries occur. In addition, the alternatives to recall are seizures, injunctions, or criminal actions. These are often accompanied by adverse publicity, which can damage a firm's reputation.

A Model Recall

Anticipatory risk planning:

- Develop a system that accurately and efficiently monitors all reports of adverse reactions
- Develop a chain of reporting
- Integrate product compliance and quality control systems
- Develop a system to track and operate customer lists
- Orchestrate a mock recall
- If there is the possibility of a recall, develop a team

Elements of a successful recall (with everything happening at once):

- Notify the FDA and identify all other applicable agencies
- Identify all customers
- Establish customer hot lines and develop a system to track
- Draft notices to physicians, distributors, and patients, if available
- Develop a team to see if anything is wrong and what went wrong
- Create a chronology
- Collect all MEDWATCH reports
- Create a team to investigate
- Implement a plan for the return of the product
- Prepare an Internet update; include an e-mail address
- Prepare for the FDA investigations and inspections as well as foreign regulatory agency requests and responses
- Identify all reporting requirements, for example, pharmaco-vigilance reports in the European Community
- Document everything

Establish priorities:

- Make the safety of the patient number one
- Immediately identify what caused the problem and then contain it
- Communicate and be active
- Tell the truth to all—no matter how bad or how good it is
- Take steps to preserve the business and the reputation of the company
- Find out what people are saying and what they are thinking

- Get the expertise you need

- Lawyers are your frontline soldiers

- Get toxicologists, a public relations expert, and a security expert

- Get the FDA involved fast and keep them advised

- Let them know what you are going to do before you do it

- Identify the lot problem and recall all of it in cooperation with the FDA

- Develop a strong relationship with the media

- Develop a strategy so that the problem is dealt with on an international basis

- Keep your insurance carriers advised—you may have a claim under your policy

- "We take the position that reasonable preventive measures that are designed to stop further injury and consequently further liability are covered by a product liability insurance policy unless specifically excluded."

Elements

Develop a written contingency plan that identifies who is responsible for directing recalls, implementing communications, and covering every aspect of the recall. Update it and redistribute it regularly.

Have an internal recall task force chaired by a top executive. It should be composed of:

- Quality control/quality assurance

- Sales

- Medical

- Legal

- Regulatory

Duties: Prepare a complete set of operating procedures

Chapter 6

Establishment Registration and Listing

R *egistration* is a process through which the owner/operator of an establishment that manufactures, assembles, or otherwise processes a device for distribution in the United States provides to the FDA information about the facility and its management.

Listing is the process that identifies to the FDA the types of devices that a firm distributes or offers for distribution in the United States.

Definitions

The following definitions are relevant to this section:

21 CFR § 807.3 (b) **commercial distribution**—any distribution of a device intended for human use that is held or offered for sale but does not include the following: 1) internal or interplant transfer of a device between establishments within the same parent, subsidiary, and/or affiliate company; 2) any distribution of a device intended for human use that has in effect an approved exemption for investigational use under section 520(g) of the act and part 812 of this chapter; 3) any distribution of a device, before the effective date of part 812 of this chapter, that was not introduced or delivered for introduction into interstate commerce for commercial distribution before May 28, 1976, and that is classified into class III under section 513(f) of the act, provided, that the device is intended solely for investigational use, and under section 501(f)(2)(A) of the act the device is not required to have an approved premarket approval application as provided in section 515 of the act; or 4) for foreign establishments, the distribution of any device that is neither imported nor offered for import into the United States.

21 CFR § 807.3 (c) **establishment**—a place of business under one management at one general physical location at which a device is manufactured, assembled, or otherwise processed.

21 CFR § 807.3 (e) **official correspondent**—the person designated by the owner or operator of an establishment as responsible for the following: 1) the annual registration of the establishment; 2) contact with the FDA for device listing; 3) maintenance and submission of a current list of officers and directors to the FDA

upon the request of the commissioner; 4) the receipt of pertinent correspondence from the FDA directed to and involving the owner or operator and/or any of the firm's establishments; and 5) the annual certification of MDRs required by Section 804.30 of this chapter or forwarding the certification form to the person designated by the firm as responsible for the certification.

21 CFR § 807.3 (f) **owner or operator**—the corporation, subsidiary, affiliated company, partnership, or proprietor directly responsible for the activities of the registering establishment.

21 CFR § 807.3 (g) **initial importer**—any importer who furthers the marketing of a device from a foreign manufacturer to the person who makes the final delivery or sale of the device to the ultimate consumer or user, but does not repackage, or otherwise change the container, wrapper, or labeling of the device or device package.

21 CFR § 807.3 (r) **United States agent**—a person residing in or maintaining a place of business in the United States whom a foreign establishment designates as its agent. This definition excludes mailboxes, answering machines, or services, or other places where an individual acting as the foreign establishment's agent is not physically present.

REGULATORY REQUIREMENT: 21 CFR PART 807 ESTABLISHMENT REGISTRATION AND DEVICE LISTING FOR MANUFACTURERS AND INITIAL IMPORTERS OF DEVICES

Establishment Registration

The requirement to register applies to both domestic and foreign firms. If an establishment is registering for the first time, it is the responsibility of the owner/operator to complete form FDA 2891 "Initial Registration of Device Establishment." Owner/operators are required to submit the initial registration within 30 days after entering into any activity requiring registration, including processing devices for exportation outside of the United States. The FDA will send an acknowledgement letter with the owner/operator identification (ID) number assigned to the firm; the assignment of the registration number will follow within 30 to 90 days. The owner/operator number can be used as proof that the registration process has been completed until a registration number is assigned.

On November 27, 2001, the FDA published the final regulation amending Part 807 to require foreign establishments to register their facilities. The regulation became effective February 11, 2002, and the FDA began enforcing these requirements April 26, 2002. Unique to foreign establishments is the additional requirement to name a U.S. agent. Until FDA form 2891(b) is available from the FDA, foreign establishments must notify the FDA in a letter signed by the official correspondent and should include the name of a person or business name, street address, telephone and fax numbers, and e-mail address of the U.S. agent. The letter must reference the foreign establishment name, address, official correspondent, and registration number. If a foreign firm is registering its establishment for the first time, FDA form 2891 should accompany the U.S. agent letter (or FDA form 2891(b) when available). FDA Form 2891 cannot be used to identify the U.S. agent.

All registration information is verified and updated annually. The FDA will automatically notify registered establishments annually with form FDA 2891(a) to verify and correct information. The form is returned to the FDA. When changes occur in ownership, establishment name, official correspondent, or address, a letter must be sent to the FDA informing them of the changes within 30 days.

The following types of establishments (domestic or foreign) are required to register:

- *Certifying site/MDR reporting site.* Registered site responsible for submission of the annual certification of the number of MDR reports submitted

- *Domestic distributor.* Any person who furthers the marketing of a device from the original place of manufacture to the person who makes final delivery or sale to the ultimate consumer or user, but does not repackage, or otherwise change the container, wrapper, or labeling of the device or device package. This category also includes, but is not limited to, direct sale, mail order, leasing, distributing promotional samples, distributing demonstration units, and drop shipping. Distributor does not include brokers or other persons who do not own the device but merely perform a service for the person (other than the ultimate consumer) who does own the device.

- *Contract manufacturer.* Manufactures a finished device to another establishment's specifications. The manufacturing establishment does not commercially distribute the device under its own name.

- *Manufacturer.* Makes by chemical, physical, biological, or other procedures, any article that meets the definition of "device" in section 201(h) of the FDCA.

- *Repackager.* Packages finished devices from bulk or repackages devices made for the establishment by a manufacturer into different containers (excluding shipping containers).

- *Relabeler.* Changes the content of the labeling from that supplied from the original manufacturer for distribution under the establishment's own name. A relabeler does not include establishments that do not change the original labeling but merely add their own name.

- *Specification developer.* Develops specifications for a device that is distributed under the establishment's own name but performs no manufacturing.

- *Contract sterilizer.* Provides a sterilization service for another establishment's devices.

- *Remanufacturer.* Any person who processes, conditions, renovates, repackages, restores, or does any other act to a finished device that significantly changes the finished device's performance or safety specifications, or intended use.

- *Initial distributor.* Takes first title to devices imported into the United States.

- *Refurbishers.* Persons who, for the purpose of resale or redistribution, visually inspect, functionally test, and service devices, as may be required, to demonstrate that the device is in good repair and performing all the functions for which it is designed. The device may or may not be cosmetically enhanced. Preventive maintenance procedures are performed. Refurbishers do not significantly change a finished device's performance or safety specifications or intended use.

- *Reconditioners.* Persons who, for the purpose of resale or redistribution, visually inspect, functionally test, and service devices, as may be required, to demonstrate that the device is in good repair and performing all the functions for which it is designed. The device may or may not be cosmetically enhanced. Preventive maintenance is not performed. Reconditioners do not significantly change a finished device's performance or safety specifications or intended use.

Device Listing

The owner/operator of an establishment that is required to list should do so within 30 days of beginning a manufacturing operation as discussed previously under "Registration Listing." This requirement applies to both domestic and foreign manufacturers. If an establishment is registering for the first time, both the Establishment Registration (FDA-2891) and Medical Device Listing (FDA-2892) must be submitted together.

An owner/operator of an establishment located outside of the United States registering for the first time must list its devices prior to exporting to the United States and the letter identifying the U.S. agent should be included. Form FDA-2892, Medical Device Listing, "Instructions for Completion of Medical Device Registration and Listing Forms FDA-2891, 2891a, and 2892" contains information on the listing process, instructions, and a sample form. The FDA has developed a product classification database to identify general categories. Form FDA-2892 is required for each general category (classification/device name) of device. Product families that carry the same product code can be listed as one product code. An owner/operator completes one form FDA-2892 for all of its establishments that manufacture the device. If the device requires a premarket notification 510(k) or premarket approval, the product code on the form FDA-2892 should be the same as that provided on the FDA clearance or approval letter unless a new product code has been created that better represents the generic device category.

Unlike establishment registration, the FDA does not issue an annual update for device listing. Owner/operators are responsible for keeping data on their listing forms current. A change to the brand or trade name of the product does not require updating the device listing. The FDA should be notified by submitting a form FDA 2892 for one or more of the following conditions indicating the changes at the time they occur:

- A "new" device is marketed with a classification name that is not currently listed.

- The intended use of a listed device changes, resulting in different general category (classification name).

- The marketing of all models or variations of the listed device is discontinued.

- A discontinued device type that is not listed is remarketed.

- Any information that was supplied on the form FDA-2892 has changed, other than changes in proprietary and common or usual name.

SUMMARY

It is important to recognize that registration and listing of an establishment is not an approval of the establishment or its devices by the FDA and does not provide FDA clearance to market. Unless exempt, premarketing clearance is required before a device can be placed into commercial distribution in the United States.

Chapter 7

Device Tracking

DEVICE TRACKING REGULATION 21CFR 821

Manufacturers must adopt a method of tracking any class II and class III devices whose failure would be reasonably likely to have serious, adverse health consequences, are intended to be implanted in the human body for more than one year, or are life-sustaining or life-supporting devices used outside of a device user facility. The statutory authority for the MDR regulation is section 519 (e) of the FDCA. The regulation 21 CFR part 821 implemented the device tracking requirements effective as of August 29, 1993. Effective February 19, 1998, the tracking requirement has been changed to eliminate the automatic mandatory tracking for certain devices.

Definitions

act—the FDCA, 21 USC 321 et seq., as amended.

importer—the initial distributor of an imported device who is required to register under section 510 of the act and Section 807.20 of this chapter. "Importer" does not include anyone who only performs a service for the person who furthers the marketing, that is, brokers, jobbers, or warehousers.

manufacturer—any person, including any importer, repacker, and/or relabeler, who manufactures, prepares, propagates, compounds, assembles, or processes a device or engages in any of the activities described in Section 807.3(d) of this chapter.

device failure—the failure of a device to perform or function as intended, including any deviations from the device's performance specifications or intended use.

serious adverse health consequences—any significant adverse experience related to a device, including device-related events that are life-threatening or that involve permanent or long-term injuries or illnesses.

permanently implantable device—a device that is intended to be placed into a surgically or naturally formed cavity of the human body to continuously assist, restore, or replace the function of an organ system or structure of the human body throughout the useful life of the device. The term does not include any device that is intended and used for temporary purposes or that is intended for explanation.

life-supporting or life-sustaining device (used outside a device user facility)—a device that is essential, or yields information that is essential, to the restoration or continuation of a bodily function important to the continuation of human life that is intended for use outside a hospital, nursing home, ambulatory surgical facility, or diagnostic or outpatient treatment facility. Physicians' offices are not device user facilities and, therefore, devices used therein are subject to tracking if they otherwise satisfy the statutory and regulatory criteria.

distributor—any person who furthers the distribution of a device from the original place of manufacture to the person who makes delivery or sale to the ultimate user, that is, the final or multiple distributor, but who does not repackage or otherwise change the container, wrapper, or labeling of the device or device package.

final distributor—any person who distributes a tracked device intended for use by a single patient over the useful life of the device to the patient. This term includes, but is not limited to, licensed practitioners, retail pharmacies, hospitals, and other types of device user facilities.

distributes—any distribution of a tracked device, including the charitable distribution of a tracked device. This term does not include the distribution of a device under an effective investigational device exemption in accordance with section 520(g) of the act and part 812 of this chapter or the distribution of a device for teaching, law enforcement, research, or analysis as specified in Section 801.125 of this chapter.

multiple distributor—any device user facility, rental company, or any other entity that distributes a life-sustaining or life-supporting device intended for use by more than one patient over the useful life of the device.

licensed practitioner—a physician, dentist, or other healthcare practitioner licensed by the law of the state in which he or she practices to use or order the use of the tracked device. (m) Any term defined in section 201 of the act shall have the same definition in this part.

Regulatory Requirement: Subpart A—General Provisions
Section 21 CFR § 821.2 Exemptions and Variances

a. A manufacturer, importer, or distributor may seek an exemption or variance from one or more requirements of this part.

b. A request for an exemption or variance shall be submitted in the form of a petition under Section 10.30 of this chapter and shall comply with the requirements set out therein, except that a response shall be issued in 90 days. The director or deputy directors, CDRH, or the director, Office of Compliance, CDRH, shall issue responses to requests under this section. The petition shall also contain the following:

   1. The name of the device and device class and representative labeling showing the intended use(s) of the device

   2. The reasons that compliance with the tracking requirements of this part is unnecessary

3. A complete description of alternative steps that are available, or that the petitioner has already taken, to ensure that an effective tracking system is in place

4. Other information justifying the exemption or variance.

c. An exemption or variance is not effective until the director, Office of Compliance and Surveillance, CDRH, approves the request under Section 10.30(e)(2)(i) of this chapter.

d. For petitions received under this section before August 29, 1993, the FDA will, within 60 days, approve or disapprove the petition or extend the effective date of this part for the device that is the subject of the petition. Any extension that the FDA grants to the effective date will be based upon the additional time the FDA needs to complete its review of the petition.

Discussion

A petition for exemption or variance to the tracking regulation may be submitted per section 21 CFR § 10.30. Any petition must be formally approved by the center prior to discontinuation of medical device tracking of any device.

Regulatory Requirement: 21 CFR § 821.4 Imported Devices

For purposes of this part, the importer of a tracked device shall be considered the manufacturer and shall be required to comply with all requirements of this part applicable to manufacturers. Importers must keep all information required under this part in the United States.

Regulatory Requirement 21 CFR § 821.20 Devices Subject to Tracking

a. A manufacturer of any device the failure of which would be reasonably likely to have a serious adverse health consequence, that is either a life-sustaining or life-supporting device used outside of a device user facility or a permanently implantable device, or a manufacturer of any other device that the FDA, in its discretion, designates for tracking, shall track that device in accordance with this part.

b. Manufacturers have the responsibility to identify devices that meet the criteria for tracking and to initiate tracking. By way of illustration and to provide guidance, the FDA has set out a list of example devices it regards as subject to tracking under the criteria set forth in this regulation.

  1. Permanently implantable devices. 21 CFR Classification

   • 870.3450 Vascular graft prosthesis of less than 6 millimeters in diameter

   • 870.3460 Vascular graft prosthesis of 6 millimeters and greater diameter, Total temporomandibular joint prosthesis, Glenoid fossa prosthesis. Mandibular condyle prosthesis, Interarticular disc prosthesis (interpositional implant).

   • 870.3545 Ventricular bypass (assist) device

- 870.3610 Implantable pacemaker pulse generator
- 870.3680 Cardiovascular permanent pacemaker electrode
- 870.3800 Annuloplasty ring
- 870.3925 Replacement heart valve, Automatic implantable cardioverter/defibrillator
- 878.3720 Tracheal prosthesis
- 882.5820 Implanted cerebellar stimulator 882.5830 Implanted diaphragmatic/phrenic nerve stimulator, Implantable infusion pumps

2. Life-sustaining or life-supporting devices used outside device user facilities. 21 CFR Classification

- 868.2375 Breathing frequency monitors (apnea monitors) (including ventilatory efforts monitors)
- 868.5895 Continuous ventilator
- 870.5300 DC-defibrillator and paddles

3. The FDA designates the following devices as subject to tracking. Manufacturers must track these devices in accordance with this part. 21 CFR Classification

- 876.3350 Penile inflatable implant
- 878.3530 Silicone inflatable breast prosthesis
- 878.3540 Silicone gel-filled breast prosthesis
- 876.3750 Testicular prosthesis, silicone gel-filled, silicone gel-filled chin prosthesis, silicone gel-filled angel chik reflux valve
- 880.5725 Infusion pumps

The FDA, when responding to premarket notification submissions and approving premarket approval applications, will notify the sponsor that the FDA believes the device meets the criteria of section 519(e)(1) and therefore should be tracked. The FDA will also, after notifying the sponsor, publish a notice in the Federal Register announcing that the FDA believes a new generic type of device is subject to tracking and soliciting comment on the FDA's position. If the device is a new generic type of device not already on the aforementioned example list, the FDA will add it to this list.

Discussion

A list of examples and specific devices that must be tracked can be found in section 821. The final decision on whether a device is to be tracked is agreed upon by the firm in conjunction with the FDA at the time of preapproval or market clearance, or in the subsequent case of a petition or variance review. This will mean that the form is required to provide a system with the means to track the control number beyond the requirements of 820.65 Traceability to the user. The tracking regulation requires traceability of the individual device to the patient with a response to the manufacturer that provides the complete and accurate information about the patient and their assigned device.

Regulatory Requirement 21 CFR § 821.25 Device Tracking System and Content Requirements: Manufacturer Requirements

a. A manufacturer of a tracked device shall adopt a method of tracking for each such type of device that it distributes that enables a manufacturer to provide the FDA with the following information in writing for each tracked device distributed:

1. Except as required by order under section 518(e) of the act, within three working days of a request from the FDA, prior to the distribution of a tracked device to a patient, the name, address, and telephone number of the distributor, multiple distributor, or final distributor holding the device for distribution and the location of the device

2. Within 10 working days of a request from the FDA for life-sustaining or life-supporting devices used outside a device user facility that are intended for use by a single patient over the life of the device and permanent implants that are tracked devices, after distribution to or implantation in a patient:

   • The lot number, batch number, model number, or serial number of the device or other identifier necessary to provide for effective tracking of the devices

   • The date the device was shipped by the manufacturer

   • The name, address, telephone number, and social security number (if available) of the patient receiving the device

   • The date the device was provided to the patient

   • The name, mailing address, and telephone number of the prescribing physician

   • The name, mailing address, and telephone number of the physician regularly following the patient if different than the prescribing physician

   • If applicable, the date the device was explanted and the name, mailing address, and telephone number of the explanting physician; the date of the patient's death; or the date the device was returned to the manufacturer, permanently retired from use, or otherwise permanently disposed of

3. Except as required by order under section 518(e) within 10 working days of a request from the FDA for life-sustaining or life- supporting devices used outside device user facilities that are intended for use by more than one patient and that are tracked devices, after the distribution of the device to the multiple distributor:

   • The lot model number, batch number, serial number of the device, or other identifier necessary to provide for effective tracking of the device

   • The date the device was shipped by the manufacturer

   • The name, address, and telephone number of the multiple distributor

   • The name, address, telephone number, and social security number (if available) of the patient using the device

   • The location of the device

   • The date the device was provided for use by the patient

- The name, address, and telephone number of the prescribing physician

- If and when applicable, the date the device was returned to the manufacturer, permanently retired from use, or otherwise permanently disposed of

b. A manufacturer of a tracked device shall keep current records in accordance with its standard operating procedure of the information identified in paragraphs (a)(1), (a)(2), and (a)(3)(i) through (a)(3)(iii) of this section on each tracked device released for distribution for as long as such device is in use or in distribution for use.

c. A manufacturer of a tracked device shall establish a written standard operating procedure for the collection, maintenance, and auditing of the data specified in paragraphs (a) and (b) of this section. A manufacturer shall make this standard operating procedure available to the FDA upon request. A manufacturer shall incorporate the following into the standard operating procedure:

  1. Data collection and recording procedures, which shall include a procedure for recording when data that are required under this part are missing and could not be collected and the reason why such required data are missing and could not be collected

  2. A method for recording all modifications or changes to the tracking system or to the data collected and maintained under the tracking system, reasons for any modification or change, and dates of any modification or change. Modification and changes included under this requirement include modifications to the data (including termination of tracking), the data format, the recording system, and the file maintenance procedures system

  3. A quality assurance program that includes an audit procedure to be run for each device product subject to tracking, at not less than six-month intervals for the first three years of distribution and at least once a year thereafter. This audit procedure shall provide for statistically relevant sampling of the data collected to ensure the accuracy of data and performance testing of the functioning of the tracking system.

d. When a manufacturer becomes aware that a distributor, final distributor, or multiple distributor has not collected, maintained, or furnished any record or information required by this part, the manufacturer shall notify the FDA district office responsible for the area in which the distributor, final distributor, or multiple distributor is located of the failure of such persons to comply with the requirements of this part. Manufacturers shall have taken reasonable steps to obtain compliance by the distributor, multiple distributor, or final distributor in question before notifying the FDA.

e. A manufacturer may petition for an exemption or variance from one or more requirements of this part according to the procedures in Section 821.2 of this chapter.

Regulatory Requirement 21 CFR § 821.30 Tracking Obligations of Persons Other Than Device Manufacturers: Distributor Requirements

a. A distributor, final distributor, or multiple distributor of any tracked device shall, upon purchasing or otherwise acquiring any interest in such a device, promptly provide the manufacturer tracking the device with the following information:

- The name and address of the distributor, final distributor, or multiple distributor
- The lot number, batch number, model number, or serial number of the device or other identifier used by the manufacturer to track the device
- The date the device was received
- The person from whom the device was received
- If and when applicable, the date the device was explanted, the date of the patient's death, or the date the device was returned to the distributor, permanently retired from use, or otherwise permanently disposed of

b. A final distributor, upon sale or other distribution of a tracked device for use in or by the patient, shall promptly provide the manufacturer tracking the device with the following information:

- The name and address of the final distributor
- The lot number, batch number, model number, or serial number of the device or other identifier used by the manufacturer to track the device
- The name, address, telephone number, and social security number (if available) of the patient receiving the device
- The date the device was provided to the patient or for use in the patient
- The name, mailing address, and telephone number of the prescribing physician
- The name, mailing address, and telephone number of the physician regularly following the patient if different than the prescribing physician
- When applicable, the date the device was explanted and the name, mailing address, and telephone number of the explanting physician, the date of the patient's death, or the date the device was returned to the manufacturer, permanently retired from use, or otherwise permanently disposed of

c. 1. A multiple distributor shall keep written records of the following each time such device is distributed for use by a patient:

- The lot number, batch number, model number, or serial number of the device or other identifier used by the manufacturer to track the device
- The name, address, telephone number, and social security number (if available) of the patient using the device
- The location of the device
- The date the device was provided for use by the patient
- The name, address, and telephone number of the prescribing physician
- The name, address, and telephone number of the physician regularly following the patient if different than the prescribing physician
- When applicable, the date the device was permanently retired from use or otherwise permanently disposed of

2. Except as required by order under section 518(e) of the act, any person who is a multiple distributor subject to the record-keeping requirement of paragraph (c)(1) of this section shall, within five working days of a request from the manufacturer or within 10 working days of a request from the FDA for the information identified in paragraph (c)(1) of this section, provide such information to the manufacturer or the FDA.

   A distributor, final distributor, or multiple distributor shall make any records required to be kept under this part available to the manufacturer of the tracked device for audit upon written request by an authorized representative of the manufacturer.

e. A distributor, final distributor, or multiple distributor may petition for an exemption or variance from one or more requirements of this part according to the procedures in Section 821.2.

Discussion

The device manufacturer shall establish the method of tracking. The method should also be well understood and implemented by the distributor(s). All associated business processes and operating systems should include the method and responsibilities to ensure that the tracking is carried forward to the user facility upon delivery of the device. The manufacturer must provide a mechanism within the system to ensure that the distributor and patient information is received back into the manufacturer quality system in a timely manner. There are detailed requirements for the manufacturer and distributor(s) to provide information within a specified time frame to the FDA regarding the device, the patient, and the physician. In the event that the distributors are remiss in carrying out their duties within the process of device tracking, the FDA will be expected to get involved to assure that the tracking information is always complete, accurate, and current. It is up to the manufacturer to notify the FDA in the event that there are any system breakdowns on the part of the distributor that cannot otherwise be resolved.

Key consideration: The most effective way to ensure that the distributors are aware of the tracking requirements is to build the requirements into the business contract with the distributor. In addition to providing the requirements in the contract, it is highly recommended that the method used to ensure device tracking through distribution is for the manufacturer and the distributor to design and agree to the process. Periodically, that system should be challenged by means of a mock recall, as well as audits of the inventory, records, and quality system.

Regulatory Requirement: Subpart D—Records and Inspections 21 CFR § 821.50 Availability

a. Manufacturers, distributors, multiple distributors, and final distributors shall, upon the presentation by an FDA representative of official credentials and the issuance of Form FDA 482 at the initiation of an inspection of an establishment or person under section 704 of the act, make each record and all information required to be collected and maintained under this part and all records and information related to the events and persons identified in such records available to FDA personnel.

b. Records and information referenced in paragraph (a) of this section shall be available to FDA personnel for purposes of reviewing, copying, or any other use related to the enforcement of the act and this part. Records required to be kept by this part shall be kept in a centralized point for each manufacturer or distributor within the United States.

Regulatory Requirement 21 CFR § 821.55 Confidentiality

a. Records and other information submitted to the FDA under this part shall be protected from public disclosure to the extent permitted under part 20 of this chapter, and in accordance with Section 20.63 of this chapter, information contained in such records that would identify patient or research subjects shall not be available for public disclosure except as provided in those parts.

b. Patient names or other identifiers may be disclosed to a manufacturer or other person subject to this part or to a physician when the health or safety of the patient requires that such persons have access to the information. Such notification will be pursuant to agreement that the record or information will not be further disclosed except as the health aspect of the patient requires. Such notification does not constitute public disclosure and will not trigger the availability of the same information to the public generally.

Regulatory Requirement 21 CFR § 821.60 Retention of Records

Persons required to maintain records under this part should maintain such records for the useful life of each tracked device they manufacture or distribute. The useful life of a device is the time a device is in use or in distribution for use. For example, a record may be retired if the person maintaining the record becomes aware of the fact that the device is no longer in use, has been explanted, returned to the manufacturer, or the patient has died.

Discussion

All record requirements under this section must be established in a formally documented system. Every point in the process where the system requires responsibility and action should be clearly defined within that system (that is, manufacturer, distributor, retailer, rental firm, user facilities, and other licensed practitioners). The outputs from that system that provide evidence of accuracy, completeness, and current status of each device and the associated patient must be available during internal audits and investigations, as well as for the FDA during site inspections. Those records and all information contained thereof will remain confidential at all times. The records should be maintained while the device is in functional use. If there is no proof that the device has been explanted, returned, or that the patient has died, then those records should be maintained.

Chapter 8

Electronic Records and Signatures

ELECTRONIC RECORDS AND ELECTRONIC SIGNATURES 21 CFR PART 11

On March 20, 1997, the FDA published a regulation in the Federal Register concerning the use of electronic records and electronic signatures.[1] This regulation defines the criteria for which the FDA considers the use of electronic records and electronic signatures as equivalent to paper records and handwritten signatures. The regulation is Title 21 of the Code of Federal Regulations (CFR) Part 11 and is effective as of August 20, 1997.

This regulation has been greatly anticipated as technology evolution allows companies to place greater reliance on electronic records. As regulatory requirements for record control and retention increase and companies strive for greater efficiency, a transition to electronic records is both a logical and necessary step.

This discussion is not meant to provide a comprehensive discussion of all elements of the regulation; it is meant to summarize key points that are required for electronic records and electronic signatures. To gain more information you can download the regulation from the Internet at fda.gov/ora/compliance_ref/part11.

SUBPART B: ELECTRONIC RECORDS

Controls for Closed Systems

The regulation states that people who use closed systems to "create, modify, maintain, or transmit electronic records" are to implement the following procedures and controls:

11.10.a. Validation of Systems to Ensure Accuracy, Reliability, Consistency, and Ability to Detect Record Changes. This regulation does not define the criteria for validation; instead, other FDA guidelines are to be used to identify what documents are applicable (such as the *General Principles of Software Validation*, Draft version 1.1, June 9, 1997, available at the FDA Web site).[2]

11.10.b. Ability to Produce Copies in Electronic and Human Readable Form. The requirement continues to state that the copies must be accurate and complete. The system must provide a capability to generate reports on the stored data for review. This has raised questions regarding the level of detail of data that is to be provided and whether the "raw" data must be maintained. The manufacturer should specifically identify the data and reports that are within the scope of this requirement.

11.10.c. Protection to Ensure Access throughout Storage Period. This means that record retention must be defined, including archival processes. Problems concerning this requirement include concerns as to whether the stored media (such as a disk) can actually be read for the duration of the retention period given the rapid evolution of technology (that is, will 5½-inch floppies be readable in available hardware 10 years from now?). The manufacturer should define a product life to clarify record retention time and also ensure that backup procedures are established.

11.10.d. Limiting System Access to Authorized Individuals. Password controls to limit access are to be provided as a minimum, and preferably physical restrictions to access as well.

11.10.e. Date/Time Stamped Audit Trails for Any Changes. This is a unique problem introduced by electronic records. How do you know that the record that is stored has not been modified? The system must provide controls to indicate when any new creation, modification, or deletion of records occurred; who is responsible for the change; and to retain the previous data. For many applications, custom modifications are required to satisfy this audit trail requirement. To ensure the required record integrity, one solution used by several companies is to store quality records on write-once CDs where changes cannot be made.

11.10.f. Operational System Checks. This requirement is defined to be "as appropriate," meaning where you can justify that this is not a needed requirement it need not apply. The intent here is that when events should occur in a particular order, operational sequence checks are to be implemented by the electronic system to enforce the required ordering. The checks could include sequences such as review order.

11.10.g. Authority Checks. These checks are to ensure that only authorized individuals are allowed to access records, hardware components, or perform controlled operations such as record modifications.

11.10.h. Device Location Checks. This is another "as appropriate" requirement. This concerns the ability to identify an individual as a result of the location of the log-on. In other words, access for selected functions may be restricted to not only certain individuals but also to the terminals that those individuals use.

11.10.i. Training of Personnel Who Develop, Maintain, or Use Electronic Record/ Electronic Signature Systems. This defines the need for procedures for use of the system, as well as training of personnel. A distinction is made in the training required for not only users but also the developers and maintainers of the system. The added emphasis on the developers and maintainers is to ensure that they understand the need to enforce security controls.

11.10.j. Written Operation Policies and Procedures That Hold Individuals Accountable and Liable. These policies and procedures are to ensure that everyone understands that the use of electronic records is to be controlled in the same manner as paper records. Falsification of electronic records is just as serious and is to be treated with the same severity as for paper records. (For electronic signature systems, the regulation further states that when electronic signatures are used, a certification is to be provided to the FDA stating that they are the legally binding equivalent of handwritten signatures.)

11.10.k. System Documentation Controls. This requirement is to ensure that the system-level documentation that includes security information such as passwords is also to be controlled to prevent potential falsification of records.

11.30 Controls for Open Systems

Procedures and controls are required to ensure authenticity, integrity, and as appropriate, confidentiality. Additional measures beyond the 11.10 requirements are expected for open systems such as document encryption and use of digital signature standards. It does not seem logical to have an open system where a company would allow access to electronic records that are subject to FDA scrutiny.

11.50 Signature Manifestations

Signed electronic records must contain: 1) the name of the signer; 2) the date and time of the signing; and 3) the meaning of the signature such as author, reviewer, or approver. This information is also to be provided with all readable forms of the electronic records that are accessible electronically or in printed form.

11.70 Signature Linking

Electronic signatures and handwritten signatures that are executed to electronic records have to be linked to the record to ensure that they cannot be copied or deleted. This requirement is to prevent the data associated with an individual's signing to be inappropriately linked to records that were not actually signed by that individual.

PART C: ELECTRONIC SIGNATURES

11.100 General Requirements

Electronic signatures have to be unique and cannot be reused or reassigned to anyone else. The uniqueness of the electronic signature is assured with the assignment of a unique user identification code, as is required for access to most established computer systems. It is also important that the identity of an individual be verified before they are allowed system access to prevent unauthorized personnel from gaining access. This is a common security practice that is used by credit card companies and banks to protect the privacy of individual accounts.

If a company has decided to use electronic signatures, a certification statement must be provided to the FDA stating that electronic signatures are intended to be the legally binding equivalent of handwritten signatures. This is to ensure that electronic signatures would be admissible in a court of law if necessary.

11.200 Electronic Signature Components and Controls

The regulation allows electronic signatures to be based on biometrics, such as fingerprints and voice recognition systems, or the entry of digital information, such as an identification code and password. For electronic signatures that are not based on biometric links both an identification code and password are required.

11.300 Controls for Identification Codes/Passwords

11.300.a. Uniqueness of Each Combined Identification Code and Password. Identification codes have to be unique. This is usually a standard function of the information technology department to ensure users have their own account.

11.300.b. Identification Code and Password Issuances Are Periodically Checked. Passwords have to be changed at some interval to ensure that if they are compromised, the compromised state is corrected over time. The regulation does not define the minimum period for changing, but any period greater than a year would not seem to be effective or reasonable. Password changes should also be checked to ensure that the user does not simply redefine the new password to be the same as the password previously in use.

11.300.c. Loss Management Procedures. Procedures must be established to disallow use of access cards or system accounts that are compromised due to loss, theft, or any other means. The procedures must allow for accounts to be reset in a manner that prevents compromising system access. These procedures may include issuing temporary access cards or resetting access passwords.

11.300.d. Transaction Safeguards to Prevent Unauthorized Use. Controls must be established for monitoring the system to detect possible intrusion into the computer systems. If an unauthorized intrusion is detected, it is to be immediately reported to the information technology department, and if additional violations occur, it is also to be reported to management. Automated checks must be implemented to be able to detect these intrusion attempts. Many companies define three failed attempts by a user to enter their password as a potential indication of unauthorized system access.

11.300.e. Initial and Periodic Testing of Devices. When physical devices are used for system access, such as a token or access card, procedures must be established to check these devices periodically to ensure that they function properly.

PART 11: COMPLIANCE POLICY GUIDE

The FDA published a Compliance Policy Guide for Part 11 (electronic records and electronic signatures) in May of 1999.[3] The Compliance Policy Guide states that decisions on whether to pursue regulatory actions against a company that is not compliant with Part 11 will be based on the following:

1. Nature and extent of deviation

2. Effect on product quality and data integrity

3. Adequacy and timeliness of planned corrective measures

4. Compliance history of the manufacturer

Although all of the aforementioned elements should be addressed, it is perhaps easiest to start with developing a plan for corrective measures. It is recommended that such a plan should address the following steps:

1. Establish corporate-level procedures that address security and record integrity requirements as defined under Part 11.

2. Assess internal systems that have applicability to Part 11.

3. Prioritize these systems as to those that are most critical for compliance with predicate regulation requirements (Part 820, Part 211, Part 58, and so on).

4. Analyze each system for Part 11 compliance using a checklist.

5. Establish an action plan to address any identified Part 11 deficiencies.

6. Establish a procedure to ensure that new systems are assessed for Part 11 applicability before implementation or purchase.

SUMMARY

The requirements for use of electronic records are not unreasonable and have been implemented cost-effectively by many companies. Companies that are using electronic records have realized increased efficiencies in the management of quality records and are expanding the role of these systems to include an increasing portion of the records mandated by the FDA quality system regulation and ISO 9001.[4]

Many commercial systems are being offered today to support electronic records and electronic signatures. It is recommended that the requirements of 21 CFR Part 11 be used to evaluate potential vendors to see how well their systems satisfy these requirements. As the use of electronic signatures adds additional requirements, most companies have elected to comply first with the electronic record elements and address electronic signature in subsequent phases of implementation.

⟐ **Endnotes** ⟐

1. 21 CFR Part 11—Electronic Records; Electronic Signatures. *U.S. Federal Register* 62, no. 54 (20 March 1977).
2. FDA. General Principles of Software Validation, Draft Guidance, version 1.1. Food and Drug Administration (FDA), Center for Devices and Radiological Health (9 June 1997).
3. FDA. Compliance Policy Guide section 160.850, Enforcement Policy: 21 CFR Part 11; Electronic records; Electronic Signatures. Food and Drug Administration (FDA), Office of Regulatory Affairs (13 May 1999).
4. 21 CFR Part 820—Quality System Regulation. *U.S. Federal Register* 61, no. 195 (7 October 1997).

Chapter 9

In Vitro Diagnostic Product Guidance

I n vitro diagnostic (IVD) products are regulated by the FDA under 21 CFR Part 820 as medical devices. The Division of Clinical Laboratory Diagnostics (DCLD) within the Center for Devices and Radiological Health (CDRH) has jurisdiction over all IVD products. The quality system regulation provides the rules under which all medical device products may be manufactured once those products have been approved. Since the quality system regulation was written for medical devices, it can be confusing when applying it to IVD products. DCLD considers guidance documents a critical tool for communicating their expectations and provides many of them for use by the IVD manufacturers. These guidance documents are not regulations, but they do provide a method by which a manufacturer may comply with the requirements of the regulations or an expectation of the agency. If the manufacturer follows the guidance, it will be compliant; if it does not follow the guidance, then it should document its decision to ensure its rationale meets the requirements or expectations. Guidance documents are both general in nature as well as product specific. They address quality system regulation compliance, and they address submission expectations.

For example, "Guideline for the Manufacture of In Vitro Diagnostic Products" provides a general overview of what IVD manufacturers must be aware of while manufacturing an IVD product. When reviewing this guidance it is obvious that of particular concern to the FDA are the microbiological conditions of the manufacturing facility. This guidance provides a method to ensure that the bioburden that a product has been exposed to during the manufacturing process will not affect the performance or the stability of the finished product. CDRH provides these guidances on its Web site. Any organization involved in the IVD business should become aware of this FDA Web site: www.fda.gov/cdrh/index.html. CDRH lists all applicable guidance documents.

FDA STANDARDS

Until recently, the FDA has not recognized standards for use by in vitro manufacturers other than the law enacted under the FDCA and its modification through later legislation. Recently, the FDA has provided an avenue for rapid clearance of IVD products if the manufacturer certifies conformance with an FDA-recognized standard. The recognized standards can be viewed on the CDRH Web site. The most important standard for an IVD manufacturer is compliance with the quality system requirements. The quality system requirement requires a manufacturer to implement written procedures to support the 17 specific elements of a quality system. These elements are discussed in chapter 2 of this book. Audits of each specific element are an essential part of managing the quality system. All quality system requirements should be audited at least annually. An effective audit program should also include a periodic audit of the entire quality system conducted by an independent certified outside auditor. This kind of program should ensure that the internal processes will withstand the scrutiny of a third-party assessor or an investigator from the FDA. Audits are also an important part of the purchasing controls element of the quality system regulation. Any audit performed for an IVD manufacturer should employ the array of guidance documents available, as well as the quality system regulation to ensure compliance to the regulations.

IN VITRO DIAGNOSTIC PRODUCTS

IVD product development, like all medical devices, must be done under a formalized design control process. Throughout this process the system must require formal design reviews. The purpose of these formal reviews is to ensure that the design of the IVD product meets the specific requirements for its intended use. A design control process should include phases as the product moves from concept through development into submission and launch. Although there are no specific requirements for when and at what points these reviews should take place, each critical step should be separated by a design review. These formal design reviews should be used to assess the success of the design in meeting the product specifications. Senior management must be part of these reviews. Reviews are traditionally done when project planning has been completed, when the product has been developed, prior to the FDA submission, and then some time after the product launch. A formal review is conducted after planning to ensure the plan is adequate to meet the design goals. The second formal review is normally done at the end of the development process and is used to ensure that the product's design meets the product requirements. The third review is normally conducted following clinical trials and after the design has been validated for its intended use. The fourth formal review is usually conducted after the product has been on the market for some time and customer feedback can be assessed. If changes are required as a result of the formal design review, a written justification for the change must be completed and approved. This change is then reflected in the support documentation for the project.

Chapter 10

Design Review Guidance

Design reviews are conducted during the development cycle of a medical device for many reasons. A primary reason is to ensure that the product meets specified requirements, which might include safety, reliability, function, compatibility, and others. Design reviews can be considered to be advisory but are also intended to identify and define areas where design requirements have not been fulfilled and where the design must be modified in order to fulfill those requirements.

Design reviews can take many forms with formality varying throughout the forms. Simple design reviews could take place with a small number of participants and focus on a specific design issue, or they could take place with cross-functional teams and focus on general issues such as preparation for a specific test or to move to another design phase.

REGULATORY REQUIREMENT

The FDA requirement for design review is stated in the design controls section of the regulation in 820.30. The FDA states, "Each manufacturer shall establish and maintain procedures to ensure that formal documented reviews of the design results are planned and conducted at appropriate stages of the device's design development. The procedures shall ensure that participants at each design review include representatives of all functions concerned with the design stage being reviewed and an individual(s) who does not have direct responsibility for the design stage being reviewed, as well as any specialists needed. The results of a design review, including identification of the design, the date, and the individual(s) performing the review, shall be documented in the DHF."

The American Society for Quality (ASQ) and the American National Standards Institute (ANSI) have published an American National Standard on Formal Design Review (ANSI/ASQC D1160-1995). That standard provides guidance on formal design reviews.

Definition

formal design review—A formal and independent examination of an existing or proposed design for the purpose of detection and remedy of deficiencies in the requirements of a design that could affect such things as reliability performance, maintainability performance, maintenance support performance requirements, fitness for the purpose, and the identification of potential improvements.

DISCUSSION

Formal Design Reviews

The process of reviewing designs should be documented and managed. *Managed* includes having a policy statement or procedure that states when, where, and who participates in design reviews. The policy should also establish the frequency of design reviews, where in the design process reviews must take place, and how to document and follow up on items identified in a design review.

There are a number of ways to define development lifecycles. A typical product lifecycle consists of phases defined as concept, design, and development; verification and validation testing; manufacturing transfer; and production. During these phases the types of design reviews will vary. The ANSI/ASQC standard describes the following design reviews:

- Preliminary
- Detailed, final
- Manufacturing
- Installation
- Use

Another type of review would be the testing review, which is also detailed and prior to manufacturing.

Preliminary design reviews are conducted to determine if the product requirements have been defined correctly and to establish the product characteristics. At this point, medical products regulatory strategies and pathways are also discussed.

Detailed design reviews are conducted to verify specific design issues such as software and hardware structure, component choices, results of testing, cost and manufacturing baselines, and to allow for the production of pilot units.

Final design reviews are to verify that all listed requirements have been met in the design or to modify the requirements or the design.

The manufacturing design review can also be called the design transfer review. At this point the reviewers are determining if all manufacturing plans that have been established are appropriate. Process validation studies would be conducted and reviewed during this phase.

Products that are installed can be reviewed after installation to ensure that requirements have been met. Products can also be reviewed during early use and periodically to ensure that the product is performing as intended.

Design Review Teams

Every review team should have specific people involved. The attendees can vary depending on the type of review and the phase, but in any case, every review should have a leader or chairperson, a secretary or note taker, and the appropriate specialists.

The FDA also requires an independent reviewer—an individual without direct experience with the product. Team members obviously must be competent, objective, and sensitive to comments and issues. The specific roles of the team members should be defined in the procedure or policy.

Planning and Scheduling

Design reviews should be planned and conducted according to a design plan. The timing of the reviews should be appropriate to the design and adjusted appropriately as project plans change. The reviews should be timed to coincide with critical decision points in a project, such as long-lead equipment purchases, regulatory submissions, clinical or other test plans, and manufacturing schedules. Preliminary reviews can take place more often if needed and deal with more specific issues.

Documentation

Every design review must have an agenda and detailed information provided to the attendees prior to the meeting in order for the review to be effective. Appropriate times are at least a week in advance wherever possible. The agenda should include the purpose of the review, the attendees, the project, the expected review time, topics reviewed, project phase being reviewed, and who will make presentations.

Results of the meeting (minutes) should be carefully documented, along with results of the review and any action items identified during the review. Any action items identified should be carefully documented and followed up on in writing or with other documentation.

Chapter 11

Risk Management Guidance

Safety risk management is a system-level requirement and cannot be isolated to software, hardware, or operational procedures. The safety risk management program must encompass a system-wide perspective that addresses all engineering disciplines and operational requirements. A comprehensive approach to a safety risk management process is defined in ISO 14971, *Medical devices—Risk Management—Application of risk management to medical devices.*[1]

RISK MANAGEMENT PROCESS

Figure 11.1 defines the risk management process. Risks are first evaluated, the level of risk is estimated, and then appropriate controls are defined to eliminate or reduce the overall safety risk. Risk controls are verified and validated as appropriate during the lifecycle development process.

ANALYSIS OF SAFETY RISKS

Analysis of safety risks is a critical first step. The earlier in the design and development process safety risks are identified, the more comprehensive the design solutions that can be provided to eliminate or reduce the risks. Although no single risk analysis method is optimum for all applications, the following list provides some of the more common and established techniques for analysis.

1. Failure mode and effects analysis (FMEA) to evaluate safety risk conditions, primarily focuses on hardware failures

2. Fault tree analysis (FTA) to examine safety risk conditions as a result of intended use conditions, environmental conditions, operator error, software errors, and integration errors

3. Hazard analysis of critical control points (HACCP) to identify process-related errors primarily associated with manufacturing processes

4. Review of complaints and recalls for similar devices to determine applicability to the current device design and operation

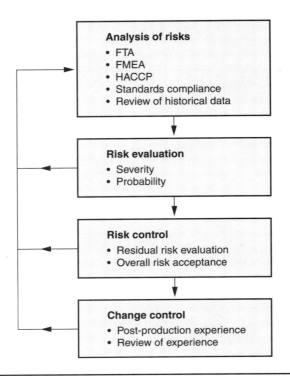

Figure 11.1 Risk management process.

5. Review of established standards and guidelines, including FDA guidelines, general requirements for medical device safety (IEC 60601-1 series standards[2]), and the Essential Requirements of the Medical Devices Directive.[3]

SAFETY RISK ESTIMATION

Decisions regarding the adequacy of safety controls are to be analyzed in accordance with a risk model. The purpose of this model is to quantify the probability and severity and ensure that appropriate safety requirements have been defined. A ranking system for defining probability and severity in a risk evaluation model is provided following.

Severity

A severity rating is defined to provide a measure of the worst credible mishap that could result should a safety mishap occur. The severity rating takes into consideration the defined safety requirements. Severity is based on a qualitative measure of the potential consequence of a safety hazard and is defined to be one of the categories, as shown in Table 11.1. These severity levels are based on criteria as defined in the Guidance for the Content of Premarket Submissions for Software Contained in Medical Device and IEC 60601-1-4.[4,5]

Table 11.1 Severity rating.

FDA Rev. Guide Description	IEC 60601-1-4 Description	Definition
NA	Catastrophic	Failures or latent design flaws could result in multiple deaths or serious injuries to the patient and/or operator
Major	Critical	Failures or latent design flaws could result in death or serious injury to the patient and/or operator
Moderate	Marginal	Failures or latent design flaws could result in non-serious injury to the patient and/or operator
Minor	Negligible	Failures or latent design flaws would not be expected to result in injury to the patient and/or operator

Probability

Probability is defined as the likelihood of occurrence over the life of the system, taking into consideration the defined safety requirements. In determining probability, the total user population, hours of operation, and system life are to be taken into account. Categories for probability of occurrence for a safety risk are defined in Table 11.2, as taken from IEC standard IEC 60601-1-4. In addition, frequency of occurrence probabilities are provided as defined in MIL-STD- 882C.[6]

Software failure modes are not like those of hardware, making specific probabilities hard to quantify. When a safety risk may be impacted by software, the probability assigned is to take into account the following:

- The level of checks and redundancy provided by the software design
- Feedback and monitoring functions
- Complexity of the software algorithm(s)

RISK CONTROL

Safety risk severity and probability are used to evaluate adequacy of risk control requirements to ensure the residual safety risk is as low as reasonably practicable. Ranking of risk severity and probability can help to identify which risks present the greatest overall risk and the necessity for additional risk control requirements. The complete evaluation of individual risks is to be used to evaluate the overall risk of the device. A diagram to be used to assess the acceptability of the overall device safety is

Table 11.2 Probability of occurrence rating.

Description	Likelihood	Probability
Frequent	Likely to occur frequently	$X > 10^{-1}$
Probable	Will occur several times in the life of the system	$10^{-1} > X > 10^{-2}$
Occasional	Likely to occur sometime in the life of the system	$10^{-2} > X > 10^{-3}$
Remote	Unlikely but possible to occur in the life of the system	$10^{-3} > X > 10^{-6}$
Improbable	Unlikely to occur during system life	$10^{-6} > X$
Incredible	Extremely unlikely to occur during system life	No probability limits defined in MIL-STD-882

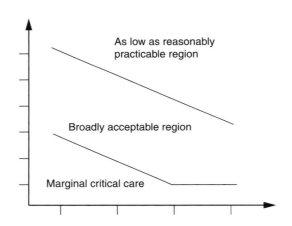

Figure 11.2 Evaluation of safety risk level.

provided in Figure 11.2. The diagram illustrates the need to reduce the risk to as low as reasonably practicable (ALARP).

All safety risks are to be tracked to system requirements and corresponding tests or labeling to ensure the effectiveness of the defined safety requirements. System requirements are to be formally tested in accordance with applicable design validation procedures. Labeling requirements are to be verified as correctly implemented in manuals, labeling, training materials, or other labeling as required.

PRECEDENCE OF ACTIONS FOR RISK REDUCTION

The preferred approach to address safety-related risks is to include system design features that preclude the occurrence of the associated events that can lead to a safety mishap. Based on the level of risk posed, other approaches may also be appropriate. System safety risk control strategies in order of preference are as follows:

1. *Design for minimal risk.* From the outset of the development process, the system design should encompass principles that eliminate or minimize the potential for safety risks.

2. *Protective measures.* If a safety risk cannot be eliminated or adequately reduced through design techniques, the safety risk should be reduced through the use of protective safety design features or methods to detect the safety-related condition and to produce a warning signal to alert personnel. Use of audio and visual alarms should be examined to determine appropriateness to the operational environment.

3. *Develop labeling, operational procedures, and provide training.* When the use of design techniques, safety devices, and warnings cannot adequately reduce the risk, labeling and training in the use of SOPs are to be applied. Tasks that have potential safety impacts require training and qualification of operations personnel.

RISK MANAGEMENT REPORT

The results of the risk management process are to be provided in a safety risk management report. The report should provide the following:

1. Identification of the safety risk

2. Description of safety risk

3. Risk control requirements

4. Severity of risk

5. Probability of risk

6. Estimation of residual safety risk

7. Mode of risk control (software, hardware, labeling, and so on) and method to verify risk control measures

Safety Risk Management Maintenance

Each manufacturer needs to have a program for evaluating device performance in the field. The evaluation program should assess customer complaints for possible safety relevance including:

1. Whether previously unrecognized hazards are identified

2. Whether the estimated risk from a previously identified safety hazard is no longer appropriate

3. Whether the original assessment is otherwise invalid

SUMMARY

A comprehensive safety risk management program is essential for the development and maintenance of any medical device. Benefits from an effective program include not only more effective design decisions but also reductions in maintenance costs, regulatory risk, and legal liability. Identification of safety risks can also support a more focused program for verification and validation activities.

☞ Endnotes ☞

1. ISO. *Medical devices—Risk Management—Application of risk management to medical devices,* ISO 14971, International Standard. 2000.
2. ANSI/AAMI ES 6060-1:2005. *Medical Electrical Equipment, Part 1: General requirements for basic safety and essential performance.*
3. Medical Device Directives. European Council Directive 93/42/EEC (14 June 1993).
4. FDA. *Guidance for the Content of Premarket Submissions for Software Contained in Medical Devices.* Department of Health and Human Services, Food and Drug Administration (May 1998).
5. International Electrotechnical Commission. *Medical Electrical Equipment, Part 1: General requirements for safety, Part 4. Collateral Standard: Programmable electrical medical systems, IEC 60601-1-4,* 1st ed. 1996-05.
6. DOD. Military Standard System Safety Program Requirements, MIL-STD-882C. Department of Defense (19 January 1993).

Chapter 12

Quality System Inspection Technique

When the quality system regulation became effective June 1, 1997, the FDA recognized the need to change their inspection method and considered a "systems approach" to evaluate a firm's level of compliance. The August 1999 document titled "Guide to Inspections of Quality Systems" was the final output from a two-year reengineering effort that changed the way the FDA conducts inspections of medical device manufacturers. The FDA recognized it was necessary to improve the efficiency and effectiveness of inspections while at the same time maximize FDA resources and reduce inspection time by conducting more focused inspections. This inspection strategy is called the quality system inspection technique (QSIT). Under the QSIT approach, an inspection should be completed within four to five days, significantly less than previous inspection times.

Often referred to as a "top-down" approach that evaluates a firm's overall ability to address quality, as opposed to a "bottom-up" approach, which begins by looking at one or more individual problems that may point to a failure in the quality system, QSIT breaks the quality system regulation into seven subsystems and directs the inspector to focus on specific elements within each subsystem considered to be key indicators that place responsibility on the firm to self-monitor compliance and to take appropriate and timely action to correct product, process, and quality system problems. The FDA concludes the inspection with an overall evaluation of the implemented quality system where management with executive responsibility is accountable to have demonstrated that they comply with the requirements of the regulation, oversee implementation, provide adequate resources, and ensure the quality system is effectively implemented and maintained.

APPLICABILITY

The FDA uses the QSIT to conduct medical device quality system/GMP inspection for both domestic and foreign manufacturers. While the "Guide to Inspections of Quality Systems" provides specific instructions for the inspector, it is designed to be used in conjunction with the following FDA policies:

- Compliance Program Guidance for Inspection of Medical Device Manufacturers (CP 7382.845)

- Investigations Operations Manual (IOM)

- 21 CFR Parts 820, 803, 804 and 821

- Compliance Policy Guides (CPG) for devices (Subchapter 300)

- Guideline on General Principles of Process Validation, FDA May 1987

QSIT inspections are preannounced inspections where the FDA will request documentation in advance to minimize the on-site inspection time. Manufacturers are under no obligation to provide the documentation; however, in the spirit of cooperation with the agency, and to minimize the disruption of an extended on-site inspection, manufacturers are encouraged to provide the documentation for the inspector to review in advance. Documentation requested in advance will be returned to the manufacturer when the on-site inspection begins.

While the primary purpose of the QSIT is for the FDA inspector, device manufacturers also use QSIT to conduct internal assessments of their quality system. QSIT does not evaluate every aspect of a firm's quality system and as a result is not considered a full quality system audit. QSIT can be an excellent tool to determine a firm's "inspection readiness" but should not be considered an alternative to, or substitute for, internal quality system audits.

SUBSYSTEMS

The FDA's Guide to Inspections of Quality Systems breaks the quality system regulation into seven subsystems with satellite subsystems under CAPA and production and process controls as applicable. The seven subsystems are as follows:

1. Management controls

2. Design controls

3. Corrective and preventive action (CAPA)

    a. Medical device reporting

    b. Corrections and removals

    c. Medical device tracking

4. Production and process controls

    a. Sterilization process control

5. Material controls

6. Records/documents/change controls

7. Facility and equipment controls

Management controls, design controls, CAPA, and production and process controls are considered the four major subsystems, as they are recognized as the basic foundation of the quality system. An evaluation of the four major subsystems will include the three remaining subsystems (materials control, facility and equipment controls, and records/documents/change controls) by their relationship to the activity or process being evaluated.

Each subsystem contains inspectional objectives, a decision flowchart, and narrative discussion for each objective. The narrative states the basic purpose/importance for the subsystem and guides the inspector through each objective in terms of the type of records to review. Links to related subsystems are noted, as well as references to specific FDA policies and compliance programs.

A QSIT inspection will begin and end with management controls. Demonstrating the top-down approach, QSIT directs the inspector to first interview the management representative (or designee) "to obtain an overall view of the management controls subsystem as well as a feel for management's knowledge and understanding of the subsystem." This interview will set the tone for the inspection. Objective 7 under management controls instructs the inspector to stop the review of the management system until the remaining subsystems have been evaluated. The order in which the remaining subsystems are reviewed is also specific: design controls, followed by CAPA, and concluding with production and process controls. Design controls and CAPA intentionally precede production and process controls, as the records and data reviewed are factors the inspector will consider when selecting a process to evaluate under the production and process controls subsystem.

SAMPLING TABLES

The "Guide to Inspections of Quality Systems" provides information for using binomial sampling plans included in the document. The inspector is instructed to select a table based on the level of confidence appropriate to the risk of the device or the records being sampled: Table 11.1—95 percent confidence or Table 11.2—99 percent confidence. While both the bottom-up and the top-down approach include a review of records, under QSIT the record review is conducted in a more controlled manner.

Chapter 13

U.S. Compliance Programs for Medical Devices

The FDA provides instructions to the field—investigators and compliance officers—through the use of compliance programs. The particular compliance program for medical devices is CPG 7382.845, Inspection of Medical Device Manufacturers—Final Guidance for Industry and FDA. This particular compliance program tells the field when to inspect medical manufacturers, what criteria to use in the inspection, what areas to look into, and what to do if the manufacturer is not compliant. It is important for industry to understand the program in order to react properly in the event of an inspection.

The document described in this section is continually being modified. The following section will generally describe the contents of each section, but it is very important that readers ensure they have the most current version and become familiar with its contents. Significant changes may occur without notification.

DISCUSSION

This section will outline each major section of the compliance program and discuss the key elements of that section:

Part I gives a general overview of the compliance program. Specifically, it discusses the cGMP regulation and describes the QSIT, it describes the MDR regulation, the medical device tracking regulation, the corrections and removals regulation, and the registration and listing regulation. Each of these is described in detail elsewhere in this book.

Part II is the implementation section. Each of the regulations is further discussed, objectives of each regulation are outlined, and inspection scheduling is described. The guidance breaks inspections into priorities, with priority A being manufacturers of high risk and class III devices and priority B being manufacturers of class II and class I devices. A priority is also given within each group starting with manufacturers that have not been inspected and following with those that have had decreasing evidence of product problems. The guidance also discusses preclearance inspections, initial inspections, routine inspections, the statutory coverage list, class I manufacturers, and follow-up inspections. Additionally, prenotification can occur in most instances where historical regulatory action has not occurred.

Part III provides the inspectional guidance for determining compliance with the quality system regulation. QSIT inspection levels are described in this section as levels 1, 2, or 3. Level one is CAPA plus one subsystem, level two is a comprehensive QSIT inspection, and level three is a compliance follow-up.

Part IV of the compliance program describes the analytical laboratories and methods to be used. The FDA has specialist laboratories across the country, and laboratories are chosen based on the type of product. The section also outlines sampling, in particular for sterility.

Part V is the regulatory section. It outlines the action to be taken in the event that the inspection has found problems. Typical regulatory actions include warning letters, however, depending on past history, injunctions, citations, detention of product, and civil penalties are possibilities. In addition, a manufacturer in this position will have premarket approvals held until resolution.

Part VI lists the contacts in the FDA for various areas. The contacts are generally considered to be used for the FDA investigators, but in the event of an issue or question, contacting the individual may be useful. Attachments to the compliance program provide other details, including lists of products affected by type of product and samples of the warning letters that are sent.

Part II
Technical Knowledge

Chapter 14

Sterilization

Confidence in the sterilization process is of ultimate importance to the manufacturer, the consumer, and to regulatory agencies. Nonsterile products, a result of sterilization process or packaging failure, have been responsible for some of the largest recalls of medical devices. The assurance of sterility may be elusive, however, due to the variables associated with a sterilization process. Process deviations during sterilization are especially significant since they have a direct and crucial impact on the safety of finished products. Therefore, regulatory agencies have required manufacturers to have a comprehensive quality assurance program that controls every aspect of the sterilization process. Such a program includes adequate environmental controls, trained personnel, maintenance and calibration of equipment, record keeping, packaging and labeling controls, and other measures applicable to the specific medical device manufacturer.

When a population of microorganisms is killed, the probability of a survivor can be calculated and may be expressed as the sterility assurance level (SAL) of the product. Most medical device sterilization processes aim for an SAL of 10^{-6}, meaning that one in a million products might be nonsterile. For products used topically on intact skin, the SAL may be 10^{-3}.

Every sterilization process must be validated, since it is impossible to test each product for sterility without destroying all the goods (such testing would be called process verification). The requirement for process validation comes from process control requirements and appears in 21 CFR 820.70, Production and Process Controls: *Each manufacturer shall develop, conduct, control, and monitor production processes to ensure that a device conforms to its specifications.* The regulation continues with specific requirements for process controls where they are needed. The remainder of Subpart G of 21CFR 820 lists requirements for control of the production environment (820.70 (c)), personnel (820.70(d)), contamination of equipment or product (820.70(e)), buildings (820.70(f)), equipment (820.70(g)), manufacturing material (820.70(h)), and automated processes (820.70(i)), as well as inspection, measuring, and test equipment (820.72). Process controls apply to sterile products at every step of the manufacturing process but in particular at the sterilization step. The *QSIT Inspection Handbook* devotes a section to the auditing of sterilization process controls. In addition, there are numerous international standards devoted to aspects of the sterilization of healthcare devices (see Methods following and references). Validation of the sterilization process indicates the resultant SAL; the sterilization process controls should guarantee the maintenance of the validated SAL.

A good validation study procedure is the beginning of the process control documentation, and it is specific for the sterilization process being studied rather than a general procedure. The study demonstrates that the process consistently results in a product meeting its specifications, which in this case includes the SAL and possibly sterilant residues and endotoxin levels. The basic elements of the study include demonstrated equipment installation performance, demonstrated process performance, and study documentation, review, and approval. The study report includes the product bioburden, the sterilization cycle parameters and tolerances, criteria for acceptance of a successful study, the process challenge studies (half-cycle runs for ethylene oxide, verification dose studies for radiation, or media fills for aseptic processing), and results of process control, monitoring, and acceptance activities (control charts, biological indicators, dosimeters). The study report provides the objective evidence that the process will consistently result in the product meeting its predetermined specifications and attributes, such as the desired SAL.

Part of the validation study includes the effect of the process on the product and its packaging. Records of post-sterilization product performance testing and packaging tests indicate that the process, and any resterilization process, does not adversely affect such characteristics as product joint strength; impact resistance; color; and tensile strength and packaging integrity, permeability, and impact resistance. Labeling resistance to moisture and temperature is also part of the study. Any materials used in the sterilization process must be reduced to specified levels and documented in the validation study (for example, ethylene chlorhydrin).

Validation studies of traditional sterilization methods are done according to recognized standards specific to the sterilization process (see references in the section Methods). If a standard is used, the requirements of the standard must be met. If the standard is not used in the validation study, there must be valid scientific rationale to support the method used in the process validation and subsequent product sterilization.

After the validation study has been approved and the sterilization cycle is in use, process controls and cycle acceptance are documented in the DHR, with each cycle being approved based on current revision procedures and cycle specifications that are part of the DMR. If the sterilization cycle is outside the tolerances for operating or performance parameters, there are procedures for handling such nonconformances and for corrective action to eliminate recurrence of the nonconformity. If a resterilization is indicated due to a process nonconformity, the effect of resterilization on the product and packaging should have been determined in the validation study in order to allow such reprocessing. Nonconformities may include positive biological indicators, high ethylene oxide residues, high bioburden, out-of-specification endotoxin (pyrogen) results, or packaging failures. Packaging failures after sterilization indicate a failure to properly validate the packaging and process combination during the original sterilization process validation (see section Packaging of Sterile Products). Periodic cycle revalidations are necessary to assure the continued adequacy of the process based on possible changes in bioburden levels, bioburden resistance, product or package changes, or equipment modifications. Purchasing and receiving of such items as sterilant, sterilization indicators, contract sterilization services, and laboratory test services are controlled by current standard procedures.

Sterilization process controls extend to the validation of the software used to control the sterilization process. If the process is automated, the software validation includes the software requirements document, the software validation protocol, software validation activities, software change controls, and software validation results to confirm that the software will meet user needs and its intended use. If the software is developed by a subcontractor, a purchasing specification and a validation report confirming that the specified software requirements were met form the minimal documentation of such a contracted software development project.

If the sterilization process is not software controlled, operating and monitoring personnel are qualified and trained to ensure a consistently successful sterilization process. Both equipment operators and quality control personnel, including those working different shifts, are trained to recognize problems that can be caused by operational errors and by not following standard procedures. Formal on-the-job training is normally required for all personnel who perform the following sterilization operations:

1. Arrange sterilizer loads

2. Place biological indicators or dosimeters

3. Manage pre- and post-sterilization packaging and warehousing

4. Calibrate and maintain sterilization and environmental control equipment systems

5. Make decisions on acceptance and rejection or need for resterilization of products

Environmental controls may also play a part in the sterilization process, depending on whether the product can be adequately cleaned before packaging. If the product cannot be cleaned, the primary production areas normally need to be environmentally controlled to minimize microbiological and particulate contamination. The amount of bacteria on the product prior to sterilization (the product bioburden) is influenced by the production environment, the handling of the product during manufacturing, cleaning processes, and hygiene of employees. The type and quantity of bacteria present on the product also influences the outcome of pyrogen testing. Pyrogen testing of finished, sterilized product will indicate if the product was contaminated with large quantities of specific bacteria (gram negative) prior to sterilization. When the bacteria are killed during sterilization, the remains of the bacteria can produce a fever (pyrogenic response) in patients under certain conditions. If the product is labeled "pyrogen free," it is important to minimize bacterial contamination prior to sterilization and to monitor finished product for pyrogen after sterilization. The end use of the product will determine whether a "pyrogen free" claim is appropriate and necessary. There are different methods of determining the presence of pyrogen so the method used to make the determination (for example, limulus amebocyte lysate [LAL]) must be detailed in the monitoring procedures. Procedures for control and monitoring of the manufacturing environment include employee gowning and hygiene, workstation cleaning and disinfection, microbiological monitoring, air filtration system maintenance, and trending of monitoring results. Any environmental monitoring program includes alert levels and action levels. The environmental specification, controls for maintaining the specification, and internal inspections are documented by the manufacturer.

Cleaning procedures are necessary to assure that microbial and particulate contamination is controlled. Changing areas and washroom facilities are provided and maintained in a clean and orderly condition; they are segregated from the production areas. Cleaning procedures for the manufacturing areas include the cleaning schedule, materials and methods to be used, and the individuals designated to perform the procedures.

Measurement and test equipment used in the sterilization process is calibrated and maintained according to specified procedures and schedules. Preventive maintenance procedures and schedules for the sterilization equipment ensure that the sterilization process parameters can be met consistently. Maintenance and calibration items to consider may include the sterilizer instrumentation, such as gages, recorder and test equipment, package sealing equipment, and cleaning of appropriate processing equipment.

Manufacturing materials required in the manufacture of sterile products may include ethylene oxide, biological indicators, incubation media, and deionized water. Each is inspected and tested for identity, viability, integrity, and purity as may be applicable to ensure the materials meet specifications. For example, when ethylene oxide is used, the manufacturer either receives certification that the gas conforms to specifications of purity and blend, or conducts tests to assure the gas meets specifications. If biological indicators are used, the performance of the bioindicators is verified by testing or certificate of analysis.

Contract sterilization is frequently used by manufacturers, but the responsibility for product sterility rests with the manufacturer, not the contractor. The manufacturer must therefore be able to produce the same documentation that would be necessary if the sterilization were being done in-house. Such documentation includes the validation study, done according to guidance from a consensus standard; process specification; product and packaging studies; procedures for cycle review and acceptance; monitoring procedures; and sterilization residual control.

Prior to release for distribution, standard procedures for testing, data, and document review, and release by a designated individual are used to ensure the finished products (lot, batch, serial number, and so on) meet acceptance criteria. The acceptance activities, including the dates of the activities, the results, the equipment used, and the signature of the individuals conducting the activities, all form part of the product documentation (DHR) required by 21CFR 820.184. The product is held in quarantine or at a controlled warehouse until it has been released for distribution. The DHR also includes the dates of manufacture, quantity manufactured, quantity released for distribution, primary identification label and labeling for each unit, and any identification and control numbers used.

The DMR of sterile products includes the specifications for the sterilizer and the sterilization process, including values for humidity, temperature, pressure, gas concentration, dwell time, conveyor speed, and so on, as applicable to the sterilization method used. There are also specifications and procedures for facility cleaning, employee dress and practices, environment, packaging, labeling, quarantine, and so on. There are instructions for performing the sterilization process, including arrangement of the sterilizer load, placement of biological indicators, identification of sterile and nonsterile product, packaging, and quarantine. Specifications for materials such as ethylene oxide and other gaseous materials, monitoring equipment such as dosimeters, media, and biological indicators are also part of the DMR. Instructions for equipment calibration, checking of charts and logs, sterility assay procedures, inspection and testing of package integrity, finished product analysis, and so on, are also required to be in the DMR per 21CFR 820.181.

Examples of sterilization deficiencies indicating that the process may not be effective include the following:

1. Abnormal percentage of lots rejected as a result of failed sterility or pyrogen tests

2. History of cycle failures, operating problems, frequent equipment breakdowns

3. Failure to properly maintain and calibrate instruments and to record such activities

4. Lack of records or incomplete records of the sterilization process and/or sterility tests

5. Failure to control the identification, segregation, and storage of finished sterile products and/or failure to control products awaiting sterility test results

6. Lack of adequate knowledge of process controls and measurement requirements by employees who operate equipment

7. Failure of the manufacturer to follow its own procedures for sterilizing products

8. Lack of specifications for the sterilization process

DEFINITIONS

absorbed dose—the quantity of radiation energy imparted per unit mass of matter. The unit of absorbed dose is the gray (Gy) where one gray is equivalent to absorption of one joule per kilogram.

aeration—the removal of ethylene oxide and its reaction products (such as ethylene chlorhydrin) from a medical device using forced warm air ventilation.

aseptic—a process in which sterile product is packaged in sterile containers in a manner that avoids contamination of the product, for example, the aseptic filling of sterile vials with sterile liquid.

batch—a defined quantity of bulk, intermediate, or finished product that is intended or purported to be uniform in character and quality, and which has been produced during a defined cycle of manufacture.

bacteriostasis/fungistasis test—a test that utilizes selected microorganisms to demonstrate the presence of substances that may inhibit the multiplication of the microorganisms.

biological indicator—a carrier inoculated with a known microorganism with a known resistance to the sterilization process under study.

bioburden—the population of living microorganisms, bacterial and fungal, on a raw material, component, finished product, or package.

calibration—the comparison of a measurement system or device of unknown accuracy to a measurement system or device of known accuracy to detect, correlate, report, or eliminate by adjustment any variation from the required performance limits of the unverified measurement system or device.

commissioning—developing the evidence that equipment has been provided and installed in accordance with its specification and that it functions within predetermined limits when operated in accordance with operational instructions.

contract sterilizer—any facility that offers to provide a contractual service intended to sterilize products that are manufactured by another establishment.

dosimeter—a device or system having a reproducible measurable response to radiation, which can be used to measure the absorbed dose in a given material.

D value—the exposure time to a sterilizing process that is required to produce a 1-logarithm or 90 percent reduction in the population of a microorganism, usually an indicator organism.

environmental controls—those controls and standardized procedures used in the manufacturing areas to control bioburden levels. Such controls may include air filters, fluid filters, use of surface disinfectants, personnel gowning or uniforms, and personnel training.

F value—a measure of the effectiveness of a heat sterilization process to inactivate living microorganisms. The F value is calculated by determining the lethal rate per minute at each process temperature using the z value of the microorganisms.

F_0 value—the F value of a heat sterilization process calculated at 121.1° C with a z value of 10 K and a D value of one minute.

installation qualification—a step in the sterilization validation program that establishes, using appropriate studies and records, that the process equipment can perform within its design specifications.

microbiological challenge—a population of known microorganisms, such as biological indicators, biological indicator test packs, or inoculated product, that can be used to test a sterilization cycle.

parametric release—a method of declaring that a product is sterile based on a review of the process data rather than on the basis of sample testing or biological indicator results.

preconditioning—a step in the sterilization process prior to exposure to the sterilizing gas mixture, designed to bring the product to specified conditions of temperature and relative humidity. This step may be accomplished within the sterilization vessel, in an external area, or in both.

process qualification—obtaining and documenting evidence that the sterilization process will produce acceptable products.

pyrogen—a biological or chemical agent that produces a fever in mammals.

sterility assurance level (SAL)—the probability of a nonsterile product after sterilization. The SAL is usually expressed as 10^{-n}.

simulated product load—A sterilization vessel load that is as difficult to sterilize as the actual product load.

sterile—free from living microorganisms. In practice, sterility is expressed as a probability function. For example, sterility may be expressed as the probability of a surviving microorganism as being one in a million (10^{-6}).

sterilization—the process used to remove all living microorganisms on a product.

sterilization dose—the minimum absorbed dose of radiation required to achieve the specified sterility assurance level.

temperature distribution study—a study to determine the temperature profile within a sterilizing chamber during a sterilization cycle.

terminal sterilization—the process in which the product is rendered free of microorganisms at the last stage(s) of the manufacturing process. In the case of ethylene oxide and radiation sterilization, the product is typically sterilized in the final packaging, including the shipping containers. In the case of moist heat sterilization, the product is sterilized in the primary container with subsequent label application and final packaging.

validation—a written procedure for developing, recording, and interpreting the data required to determine that a process will consistently yield product that complies with established specifications. In the case of sterilization cycles, validation includes commissioning (demonstrating that the equipment to be used conforms to specifications) and performance qualification (demonstrating that acceptable product will be produced when the commissioned equipment is used in accordance with documented procedures).

verification—evaluation to assure current operation or applicability for use of a system. For example, although a set of thermocouples have been calibrated, a single-point check of the thermocouples in the temperature range to be measured is considered a verification of the correct functioning of the equipment prior to and after use in developing a sterilization cycle. In other words, it is a confirmation that specified requirements have been met.

z value—the number of degrees of temperature required for a 1-logarithm change in the D value. A z value can be obtained from a thermal resistance curve; D values are plotted against temperature, and the reciprocal of the slope is determined as the z value.

METHODS

The methods used to sterilize medical devices fall into two general categories—traditional and nontraditional.

Traditional Methods of Sterilization

Dry Heat Sterilization. This method is used to sterilize heat-stable items, such as glassware and tools. This method is not widely used in medical device manufacturing because of the high temperatures involved. It may be used in aseptic production for sterilization and depyrogenation of glassware, such as vials, prior to filling. Requirements for this method may be found in AAMI ST50, *Dry Heat (Heated Air) Sterilizers,* and in prEN 866-6, *Biological systems for testing sterilizers and sterilization processes—Part 6: Particular systems for use in dry heat sterilizers.*

Ethylene Oxide (EtO) Wherein Product Is Sterilized in a Fixed Chamber. This method is a widely used process for sterilizing medical devices. Although EtO gas is toxic, flammable, and explosive, and the process leaves EtO residuals that must be removed from the product by controlled aeration, the process has several appealing traits. The equipment used is relatively affordable and the installation and operational validation process is well-documented and straightforward (ISO 11135, *Validation and routine control of ethylene oxide sterilization*). The process involves multiple variables, including EtO gas concentration, temperature, relative humidity, and exposure time, all of which must be controlled to within the limits specified during the process validation. The process usually has little detrimental effect on the materials or product being sterilized. The negative aspect of the process is the gas itself and the effect it can have on sterilizer operators and product handlers. The residual EtO and ethylene chlorhydrin are evaluated using such recognized standards as ISO 10993-7, *Biological evaluation of medical devices—Part 7: Ethylene oxide sterilization residuals*. Control of the outgassing area used to aerate products and the liability associated with employee exposure to EtO has resulted in numerous contractors who specialize in EtO sterilization of large quantities of medical products (see AAMI TIR14, *Contract sterilization for ethylene oxide*). Be aware that changing EtO sterilization contractors will require a revalidation of the cycle to assure that microbial lethality is not affected by differences between the two facilities.

A review of pertinent standards related to EtO sterilization will help one become familiar with detailed requirements for control of the process. For example, when establishing a sterilization facility, AAMI TIR15, *Ethylene oxide sterilization equipment, process considerations and pertinent calculations*, is helpful in specifying the equipment to be purchased and in calculating such important parameters as percent relative humidity and EtO gas concentration. For detailed information concerning EtO residuals testing, refer to ISO 10993-7 and AAMI TIR19, *Guidance for ISO 10993-7*. Product bioburden determination and monitoring methods can be found in ISO 11737-1, *Microbiological methods— Part 1: Estimation of population of microorganisms on products*. Also, ISO 11737-2, *Microbiological methods—Part 2: Tests of sterility performed in the validation of a sterilization process*, provides essential information for required sterility testing. Biological indicators, used in the validation and subsequent process control of EtO sterilization, are subject to the requirements in ISO 11138-1, *Sterilization of healthcare products—Part 1: Biological indicators*. Other standards that apply to EtO sterilization of medical devices include EN 550, *Sterilization of medical devices—Validation and routine control of ethylene oxide sterilization*, and EN 556, *Sterilization of medical devices—requirements for terminally sterilized medical devices*. The *FDA QSIT Inspection Handbook* sections devoted to sterilization process control provide a systematic approach to conducting an audit of sterile medical products, especially ones sterilized by ethylene oxide.

Steam. This method is more widely used to sterilize pharmaceutical and parenteral drug products, but it is also used to sterilize liquids and equipment for aseptic filling and for diagnostic products. Steam is the preferred method for sterilizing heat-stable implants, such as orthopedic implants and mechanical heart vales, and the instruments used for surgical procedures. The process involves the control of two basic parameters: time and temperature. The relationship between the two variables and their lethal effect on microorganisms is expressed by such terms as D value, F value, z value, and F_0 (see definitions at the beginning of this chapter). Requirements for validation and control of moist heat sterilization, which includes saturated steam and air-steam mixtures, are found in such standards as ISO 11134, *Requirements for validation and routine control— Industrial moist heat sterilization*, AAMI TIR13, *Principles of industrial moist heat sterilization*, and EN 554, *Sterilization of medical devices—validation and routine control of sterilization by moist heat*. Other regulatory and technical requirements may also apply to the steam sterilization of pharmaceuticals. A review of the standards will detail the information expected of manufacturers who sterilize products using moist heat.

Radiation (Gamma or Electron Beam). A method of sterilizing products, by batch or continuous processors, using radiation from Cobalt 60 or Cesium 137 or using a beam from an electron or x-ray generator. Once medical product manufacturers became aware of the disadvantages of EtO sterilization, such as the toxic effects of EtO on operations personnel, attention was focused on radiation sterilization as an alternative to EtO. Radiation has the advantage of only one process variable, time of exposure to the radiation source. However, the materials used in product and packaging design are crucial. Radiation has a deleterious effect on certain materials, such as Teflon, and can discolor materials that do not otherwise degrade. Changes in material impact strength, hardness, color, elasticity, and other performance characteristics may occur immediately or over time after radiation. Selection of radiation-stable materials is based on years of experience and testing that have been distilled into published guidance documents, including AAMI TIR 17, *Radiation sterilization—Material qualification*. After the selection of radiation-stable materials, a program involving the testing of products for all essential properties throughout the expected shelf life follows a determination of the maximum radiation dose expected. ISO 11137, *Requirements for validation and routine control—Radiation sterilization*, and EN 552, *Sterilization of medical devices—Validation and routine control of sterilization by irradiation,* are excellent guidance documents to the requirements for validation and control of radiation sterilization processes.

Radiation sterilization is dependent on the product bioburden, which is characterized during the validation study. Environmental controls and product bioburden monitoring receive more emphasis when the calculation of the radiation dose is directly related to the average product bioburden and the expected SAL. This is the method used to set the sterilization dose in Method 1 of ISO 11137. The standard includes two additional methods of dose setting, as well as somewhat complicated calculations used in each method. Application of ISO 11137 should be left to knowledgeable and experienced individuals to assure proper interpretation of the standard and the nuances involved in this method of sterilization. An alternative is to use AAMI TIR13409, *Substantiation of 25 kGy as a sterilization dose for small or infrequent production batches*. The TIR is a formalization of the old "overkill" approach to radiation sterilization wherein product was considered sterile if the absorbed dose was 25 kGy. The product must have a demonstrated average bioburden of less than 10^3 viable organisms (colony forming units or CFUs) and must be manufactured in small quantities (less than 1000 units). Radiation sterilization is usually performed by contractors who have invested in an expensive processing facility and who have a vested interest in assuring that the sterilization dose for each product is set according to recognized standards and regulations.

The real advantage of radiation sterilization is the one process variable, absorbed dose. Monitoring of a validated process involves the use of dosimeters to determine absorbed dose at various points in the product load. It is important that the loading configuration be consistent and that dosimeters be placed as specified in the load. After using the dosimeters to determine that the absorbed dose meets the cycle specification, the product may be released for distribution without delay.

Nontraditional Methods of Sterilization

1. Ethylene oxide in which EtO is injected into a porous polymer bag ("bag method," "diffusion method," "sterilization pouch," "injection method")

2. Ethylene oxide in which less common process indicators are used, such as:

   a. A long gas dwell time (more than eight hours) or the absence of a specified dwell time

   b. Use of EtO volume instead of concentration

   c. Mention of EtO (gas) cartridge

   d. Use of humidichips

   e. Use of "100 percent EtO in-house"

3. High-intensity light

4. Chlorine dioxide

5. Ultraviolet light

6. Gas plasma

7. Vapor systems (for example, peroxide or peracetic acid)

8. Filtration methods

9. Liquid chemical sterilization or high-level disinfection as the terminal process

   A new method remains a nontraditional method unless and until:

   a. The FDA/CDRH evaluates the validation data for the method of sterilization as part of a quality system evaluation and finds it satisfactory for that general type of device

   b. The specific sterilization method is incorporated into a new or existing voluntary consensus standard formally recognized by the FDA

There is a recognized standard for the validation and control of sterilization by liquid chemical sterilants, ISO 14160, *Sterilization of single-use medical devices incorporating materials of animal origin—Validation and routine control of sterilization by liquid chemical sterilants*, but it is specific to medical devices incorporating materials of animal origin. Users of the aforementioned nontraditional methods should realize they are using methods that are outside the scope of specific FDA/CDRH-recognized standards and should be prepared with a thorough and well-documented process validation study. The study does not necessarily need to be submitted to the FDA in the 510(k) application, but the FDA may decide inspection of the sterilization facility is a priority.

PACKAGING OF STERILE PRODUCTS

Packaging of sterile products is important to ensure that a safe product arrives intact (sterile) at its end user and that the product remains sterile throughout the specified shelf life and storage conditions. When a product is recalled because of a sterility issue, it is usually the packaging that has been compromised, not the sterilization process. Like sterilization, packaging operations are validated in a manner consistent with the requirements for process controls. The packaging materials and design are also validated to assure the integrity of the unit before distribution (is the packaging appropriate for the sterilization method used?) and during transit and storage. The permeability of the package to the sterilant, suitability of closures and variability associated with material finish, thickness, and composition are design factors to be considered. The sterilization cycle may compromise the effectiveness of the packaging design.

Packaging design depends on the sterility claim: either the product is entirely sterile or only the fluid path is sterile. In the first case, the packaging consists of: 1) a primary package (which may have two layers) containing the product; 2) a secondary package containing one or more primary packages to facilitate storage and internal transport by the user; and 3) a transport package to protect the product(s) during external transit from the manufacturer or distributor to the user. In the second case, where the claim is for fluid path sterility only, the secondary and transport package are sufficient, given that there are closures and fittings, to keep the inside of products sterile, that have been validated at least to the standards of the primary package.

Design of packaging that protects the product may be contradictory to ease of product sterilization. Compromises may need to be made in materials and packaging design, possibly involving further packaging operations after sterilization. For example, packaging for EtO sterilization must be permeable to the sterilant gas, but it must also be able to "breathe" at a rate fast enough to prevent seal or film failure during the vacuum steps at the beginning and end of the cycle. Yet the material must not be so permeable that it fails to protect against contamination. A compromise design may involve an impermeable plastic film primary package with an air filter "port" that allows easy flow of air in and out of the package without risk of product contamination.

As with the sterilization process, packaging is validated according to a documented study protocol to establish that the packaging process will consistently yield product that meets the specifications. ISO 11607, *Packaging for terminally sterilized medical devices*, and EN 868-1, *General requirements and test methods, packaging materials and systems for medical devices*, detail the requirements to be met when validating a product/package combination. The validation study begins with the packaging materials, which are evaluated for such properties as microbial barrier, toxicity, physical and chemical properties, compatibility with the sterilization process to be used, forming and sealing characteristics, and shelf-life limitations. Characteristics of the chosen materials are specified according to standard requirements, as listed in ISO 11607, and requirements specific to the product and the packaging and sterilization process. General material requirements include such characteristics as "free of holes, cracks, or tears," "non-leaching and nontoxic," and such physical properties as tensile strength, thickness variation, tear resistance, burst strength, and chemical properties such as pH, chloride, and sulfate content. Additional requirements may apply to adhesive-coated materials, formed packages, and reusable containers. AAMI TIR22, *Guidance for ISO 11607*, provides guidance in the choice of materials and in the use of standardized test methods to satisfy the ISO 11607 requirements. For example, ASTM F-1608 is the suggested method for testing microbial barrier properties. Tests suggested include methods for accelerated aging, gas transmission, oxygen transmission, tensile strength, tear resistance, odor, pH, wet strength, porosity seal strength, and burst strength.

After the packaging materials have been chosen, the packaging is validated for compatibility with the sterilization process and the product. Variability in the packaging materials during routine supply is a consideration. Likewise, product mass, sharp edges, and chemical interactions between product and packaging are considerations. Labeling is part of the packaging and the validation study. Labeling, including adhesives and inks, should not be affected by the sterilization process or subsequent transport and storage. Microbial barrier properties of porous and impermeable materials are characterized. Finally, the transport and storage conditions of the packaging are validated, usually by a combination of real-time and accelerated shelf-life studies. The accelerated aging protocol can be developed using guidance contained in AAMI TIR17, *Radiation sterilization—Material qualification*. Validation of transport conditions may involve testing the packaging at the maximum and minimum transport temperatures, low atmospheric pressure (high altitude), high relative humidity, controlled drop, and extended periods of vibration (affectionately known as "shake, rattle, and roll" testing).

Package forming and sealing is also part of the packaging validation study. The equipment used in forming and/or sealing is validated to document effectiveness in meeting operating limits and tolerances consistently. The equipment qualification includes the ability to monitor key parameters, calibration and maintenance procedures, inspection of tooling, cleaning procedures, software validation (if applicable), and operator training. The process development proceeds with studies to establish the upper and lower processing limits, including such parameters as temperature, pressure/vacuum, dwell time, energy levels (radio frequency), and torque limits. The process limits are challenged during a process verification study in which packages are produced at the upper and lower parameter limits that result in packages meeting specifications. In other words, the upper and lower limits of the forming parameters are used to produce packages that are inspected to determine if the packages meet dimensional requirements such that the product fits into the package and the package fits into the sealing machine and the secondary package. For the sealing process, packaging is inspected for seal width, punctures or tears, channels or open seals, and material delamination or separation. Finally, a process performance qualification study is used to document effectiveness and reproducibility of the process in multiple production runs. Established procedures for machine setup, sealing and forming process parameters, test methods for seal width, continuity and integrity, and process start-up are used during the study. Essential process parameters are monitored during the study. Results of the study are summarized and used as the process certification package. Any change in equipment, product, packaging materials, or process that may change the original validation and affect the sterility, safety, or efficacy of the product will result in the need to revalidate the affected processes.

After the packaging process has been validated, routine package inspection is used to determine if specifications are being met on a lot-to-lot basis. A sampling scheme is developed and methods for visual inspection, seal/closure evaluation (tensile seal strength test, burst/creep pressure test), and physical testing (internal pressure test, dye penetration test, vacuum leak test) are implemented. Testing is usually performed after sterilization to ensure compatibility between the packaging and the sterilization process.

An ongoing program of packaging evaluation is implemented to monitor package integrity during handling, distribution, and storage. Analysis of test data from this program will determine if further limits are necessary on the handling, distribution, and storage of the product.

A review of ISO 11607 and AAMI TIR22 is essential prior to auditing a sterile medical product packaging operation. AAMI TIR22 provides a wealth of background information to be used in the implementation of ISO 11607. The TIR is also a good source of the description of the various test methods, such as the dye penetration test.

Chapter 15

Biocompatibility

Biological evaluation of medical devices is called biocompatibility testing and is performed to determine the potential toxicity resulting from contact of the component materials of the device with the body. The testing is aimed at proving that the materials will not cause any adverse local or systemic effects, will not be carcinogenic, and will not cause any reproductive or developmental effects. The international standard for biological evaluation of medical devices is ISO 10993, which has 16 parts that deal with various aspects of such testing. Part 1 of the standard, "Evaluation and Testing," is the framework for choosing the necessary tests based on the nature, degree, frequency, and duration of exposure of the device to the body. Absolute adherence to the suggested test matrix in the standard is not essential because of such factors as the design of the device and a successful history of the materials in similar devices. If a device is made of materials with a long history of safe use and which have been well characterized in the published literature, it may not be necessary to conduct all the tests suggested in the standard.

The structure used in ISO 10993 for the selection of tests is based on the following scheme:

I. Nature of body contact: devices that contact the body fall into one of three categories:
   A. Surface contacting, in which case the device may contact:
      1. Intact skin only
      2. Mucosal membranes
      3. Breached or compromised surfaces, such as ulcers, burns, and so on
   B. External communicating, in which case the device may contact:
      1. Blood path indirectly, such as in the case of solution administration sets
      2. Tissue/bone/dentin
      3. Circulating blood
   C. Implanted devices, which may be in contact with:
      1. Tissue (pacemakers or breast implants)
      2. Bone (orthopedic implants)
      3. Blood (heart valves or pacemaker leads)

II. Duration of contact: the time the device is in contact with the body
    A. Limited (less than 24 hours)
    B. Prolonged (more than 24 hours but less than 30 days)
    C. Permanent (more than 30 days)

After the device has been properly categorized using the aforementioned scheme, the recommended tests are chosen from the tables found in the standard. The standard lists the suggested tests with a short description of each. The tests include cytotoxicity, sensitization, irritation, intracutaneous reactivity, systemic (acute) toxicity, subchronic (subacute) toxicity, genotoxicity, implantation, and hemocompatibility in the primary matrix. The secondary matrix of tests that may be considered includes chronic toxicity, carcinogenicity, reproductive and developmental toxicity, and biodegradation. Pyrogen testing is not listed and should be considered if the device may contain chemical components that may be pyrogenic. Likewise, additional tests not included in the standard may be required depending on the possibility of specific target organ toxicity. The rationale for the tests chosen, or not chosen, should be documented in a comprehensive materials test plan.

The flexibility inherent in the standard has resulted in the FDA publishing Blue Book Guidance Memorandum #G95-1, in which a modified matrix is presented that includes optional tests to be considered. For example, ISO 10993 would not require acute toxicity, subchronic toxicity, chronic toxicity, and implantation tests for a surface device permanently contacting mucosal membranes, such as an IUD. In the FDA guidance matrix, all these tests are listed as optional for surface devices that are in permanent contact with mucosa. It is therefore important to not only review the FDA guidance document prior to selecting a testing plan, but it is also advisable to consult with the appropriate FDA review division in the Office of Device Evaluation, CDRH, prior to initiating tests of any new device materials. Failure to do so can result in unnecessary, expensive, and time-consuming tests.

Biocompatibility testing is part of the overall medical device quality management plan and as such may require that materials be retested, based on changes in the product design, source of materials, or device indications.

Chapter 16

Controlled Environments and Utility Systems

Controlled environments may be required in the manufacture of medical devices depending on the application of the device. Controlled environments are typically used to ensure that the product being produced is not contaminated by environmental conditions. Those conditions can include particulate matter that adheres to the device that is not viable or living, particulates that are viable (bacteria), and other contaminates that may be chemical or process related.

Controlled environments may also be required if processing conditions require that the environment be maintained within certain ranges. Those ranges can include temperature and humidity and may also include other conditions.

It is most important to note that the controlled environment is product dependent. The product characteristics must be taken into account in any establishment of conditions for the environment. The environment can then be tested and validated to ensure that it meets the requirements.

REGULATORY REQUIREMENT

No specific regulatory requirement for medical devices is stated in U.S. or international regulations. The requirement is product dependent. However, two standards do discuss "cleanrooms." Those standards are Federal Standard 209E, Airborne Particulate Cleanliness Classes in Cleanrooms and Clean Zones, and International Standard ISO 14644-1, *Cleanrooms and associated controlled environments*. Those standards are excellent references for the establishment and control of environments.

Discussion

Cleanrooms can be classified according to the amount of particulate matter present. Particles can be liquid or solid in order to be counted. Cleanrooms can be classified as Class 1 to Class 100,000. Depending on the class, the quantity of particles of different sizes varies and can be determined by referring to tables contained in the reference standards. For example, a Class 100,000 cleanroom cannot contain more than 100,000 particles of 0.5 micron or greater per cubic foot, and 700 particles of 5 micron or greater per cubic foot.

For medical purposes, the controlled environment is a combination of requirements. The particulate cleanliness is usually stated as described in the previous paragraph, but the other conditions must be stated also.

In order to establish the environmental conditions, an initial study is done prior to using the controlled environment. In that initial study, the following conditions are considered:

- Pressure differential between the room and outside areas

- Efficiency of filtering media

- Volume of air flowing into the space

- Air changes per period of time in the space

- Aerobic and anaerobic effects

Following the initial study, the room is also studied under typical use conditions to ensure that the room continues to meet requirements. Periodic monitoring and maintenance of the control equipment is essential to ensuring that the controlled environment meets its requirements.

UTILITIES

Each controlled environment or other manufacturing area may also contain a number of utilities used to control or run equipment and the environment. Typical utilities include:

- Heating, ventilating, and air conditioning (HVAC)

- Electrical power

- Emergency electrical power

- Clean water systems

- Compressed air

- Oil and particulate controlled compressed air

Each of these utilities must be specified and tested in a similar manner to the controlled environment.

FACILITY QUALIFICATION

In order to ensure that each controlled environment and utility meets its requirements, a facility qualification is performed. That qualification begins with the development of a master plan that describes the activities and specifications. The master plan will describe a combination of protocols that are executed to determine if each system functions as intended. Protocol can consist of installation qualification, operational qualification, and performance qualification.

Chapter 17

Software

There are essentially two classes of software and two levels of software validation as defined by FDA guidelines. The first includes all software that is used by a medical "device." This category includes any devices that require submission of a 510(k) or PMA to the FDA prior to marketing. Software in this category has to be validated in accordance with the design control requirements of the quality system regulation.[1] The FDA has provided specific guidance for validation of this class of software in the Guidance for the Content of Premarket Submissions Software Contained in Medical Devices.[2]

The second category of software is any software that is used to support production of a device or implementation of quality assurance procedures. This software also must be validated "for its intended use" as defined in section 820.70(i) of the FDA Quality System Regulation. This includes any software used in the manufacturing process, such as programmable logic controllers (PLC) and manufacturing resource planning (MRP) software. In addition, any software used to support quality system requirements such as complaint tracking, failure investigation, DMRs, or DHRs also requires validation under this category. The level of validation required by the FDA for this class of software is less stringent than that required for software that is internal to a device.

SOFTWARE DEVELOPMENT PROCESS

A high-level diagram of the software development process as mapped to the elements of design controls is shown in Figure 17.1. This figure illustrates that software is like any other engineering discipline and benefits from the same up-front development activities such as reviews and testing.

REQUIREMENTS DEFINITION

The purpose of the requirements definition phase is to define and analyze the functions, interfaces, and other constraints applicable to the system. This is the most important phase of the software development process because it not only defines what the software is to do, but it also defines the basis for how the software is to be tested

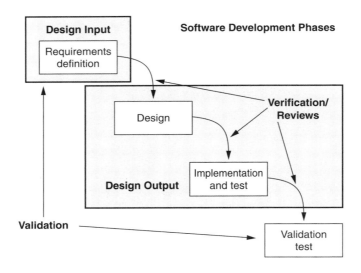

Figure 17.1   Software development process.

(the requirements are used as the basis for defining the test procedures used for validation). The following are analyzed during this phase:

1. Definition of the requirements in a manner to support ease of understanding and presentation to the customer

2. Identification of potential safety risks through the conduct of a risk analysis

3. Definition of interface requirements for interfacing hardware and/or software components, including required inputs, outputs, and constraints

A requirements specification and safety risk analysis is developed for the system during this phase. A review including the customer should be conducted to verify the correctness of these documents.

DESIGN

The purpose of the design architecture phase is to identify an optimum architecture for implementation of the requirements. During this phase, the following activities occur:

1. Alternative design approaches are analyzed and trade-off studies are performed to select the optimum design architecture. The design architecture should be depicted using a graphical notation.

2. Implementation algorithms and interface formats for hardware and software components are specified.

A design description is developed to describe the design architecture. Supplemental design studies and supporting implementation history information are documented, as applicable. Peer reviews of the design architecture are conducted to verify the quality of the design and implementation strategy.

IMPLEMENTATION

During implementation each software unit is coded and verified as correctly implemented. Prototypes are prepared to demonstrate effective system operation. During this phase, the following activities occur:

1. Software program units are coded in accordance with established programming guidelines.

2. Unit testing is performed to verify correctness.

3. Unit testing for program units that satisfy safety requirements is formally documented.

4. Code reviews are performed as directed by the project manager.

Program source code is placed under configuration management at the completion of unit testing and code reviews. System prototypes may also be produced during this phase. Design and requirements specifications are updated to reflect changes and the results of testing.

VALIDATION TEST

The purpose of the software validation test is to demonstrate that specified requirements are satisfied. System validation test procedures are to be maintained and used for retesting as required throughout the maintenance phase. During this phase, the following activities are to occur:

1. Testing is conducted in accordance with the system validation test procedures to verify satisfaction of requirements. Control of the test environment and procedures is maintained to provide a baseline for future testing.

2. Tests are conducted to ensure satisfaction of user needs and intended uses.

3. Tests are conducted to demonstrate that identified safety risks have been successfully eliminated or mitigated. Stress testing is conducted to verify safe program operation and performance under maximum loading and worst-case scenarios.

4. Testing is to include initial production units under defined operating conditions, as applicable.

5. Testing is to include actual or simulated use conditions, as applicable.

6. Discrepancy reports are generated for any defects that remain after completion of system validation testing.

7. Regression testing is performed as changes are made to ensure that the integrity of the baselined system is not affected.

8. A test summary report is generated to document the results of the test process, including a traceability matrix to demonstrate the completeness of the test program and to ensure that all specified requirements are tested.

9. Formal documentation (requirements, risk analysis, design, test, and so on is updated and prepared for delivery.

10. Operations and support documentation are reviewed to ensure that they are accurate and adequately address operation and support requirements.

DESIGN TRANSFER

Software products to be distributed on electronic media such as floppy disks or CD-ROM are distributed with an install program that will verify the integrity of all distribution files. Software products distributed on solid-state media, such as flash or EEPROM that may be embedded in a distributed device, will conduct a self-test of the program integrity to ensure that each copy is correct.

DESIGN RELEASE

Design release approval is to include review of all developed documents to verify completeness and consistency. Reviews are to include participation by an individual who does not have direct responsibility for the development activity.

ENGINEERING CHANGES

During the maintenance phase, continuing engineering and programming support is to be provided for operational programs. The maintenance activities comprise previously defined engineering phases (from requirements analysis through system validation testing) that are to be performed as a project is modified.

Delivered software is to be maintained under version control. Every product change involves updates to documentation as well as the software. The specific documents that require update are determined by the extent of the changes made and regulatory requirements. As a minimum, a history record shall be maintained to track changes made, the reason for the change, version numbers, and documentation updates. Use of an automated configuration management tool to track program change history is recommended.

The number and type of reviews to be conducted for maintenance changes is determined by the extent of the modification. Reviews shall be conducted to ensure that the changes have been successfully implemented, that the appropriate documentation has been updated, and, for safety-related changes, that safety-related test procedures are executed.

HOW TO VALIDATE PROCESS SOFTWARE

A slightly different emphasis is placed on validation of software that supports automated manufacturing and implementation of quality assurance practices. In this case validation requires, as a minimum, a requirements definition, code, and testing documentation, but does not mandate the same level of detail that is required for product software. As in the device software, the depth and detail of the documentation should be in proportion to the complexity of the application. The program areas that have the greatest safety risk should receive a more comprehensive validation focus than other areas. Programs that have a lesser effect on the safety of the product, or are verified through subsequent inspection, require less stringent validation. In all cases, the level of validation must be documented.

The fact that process software may be purchased off the shelf or developed by a subcontractor adds another dimension to the validation effort. The validation program for third-party software should again be focused on areas that present the greatest potential for risk. A close vendor working relationship and vendor certification programs can help in gaining confidence in the quality of the supplied software. If possible, the validation effort should provide visibility into developer procedures and product documentation. For proprietary reasons one may not be able to gain access to such documentation.

There is a wide range of activities that can be applied to support third-party validation. The appropriate mix of these activities is dependent on the function and risk of the software program. A list of some of the activities that can be applied to support validation of third-party software is shown in Table 17.1. Documentation must be kept to demonstrate the validation activities that were performed.

Table 17.1   Third-party software validation activities.

Testing Activities

• Functional testing to verify satisfaction of requirements

• Safety hazard analysis tracking and definition of safety testing

• Failure mode and stress testing

Review Activities

• Review of developer product specifications

• Review of developer SOPs

• Review of the results of validation activities such as programmer walk-through and inspections

Monitoring Activities

• Participation in requirements and design reviews

• Monitoring of various levels of test

• Monitoring validation activities

Management Activities

• Establish a third-party certification program

• Maintain frequent communication with subcontractors during development

• Establish a database of vendor quality characteristics

GUIDELINES FOR A SUCCESSFUL SOFTWARE DEVELOPMENT PROGRAM

The FDA guidelines for implementation of software may seem overwhelming at first, but they do provide for a great deal of flexibility. These guidelines are based on proven techniques that emphasize design engineering early in the development process. These techniques have been demonstrated to result in increased reliability and productivity as a result of less time spent in program testing and debugging. The FDA's stated objectives of product safety and effectiveness are also consistent with good business practices. The following is a list of the factors that lead to most likelihood for success of software implementations:

1. Define internal procedures for conduct of a software development process, including standards for writing specifications, guidelines for how to validate process software, and forms for identifying and tracking safety risks.

2. Foster a team development environment, including frequent communication between programmers, quality assurance/testers, and target customers.

3. Manage requirements to ensure clear understanding up front of customer needs and to prevent unwanted requirements "creep" during the development process.

4. Recognize the intent of the FDA definition of levels of concern and define a validation program that focuses additional resources on critical areas.

5. Ensure that the development process allows for early and frequent reviews and testing of the quality of the developed software. Process audits are also helpful in identifying potential problems early in development phases.

6. Use automated tools where possible to facilitate the development process, including documentation tools, tools to help trap for hard-to-find software errors, and automated test tools.

7. Establish a documentation strategy that minimizes effort by emphasizing quality over quantity through adherence to defined guidelines and effective review techniques.

8. Update software development procedures based on lessons learned from previous efforts through the definition of documentation templates, measurement tools, and checklists to increase effectiveness.

9. Provide procedure compliance and "best practices" training to all personnel associated with the development process, including developers, testers, and project managers.

10. Establish process measures to evaluate progress and monitor quality of software code and associated documents during the development process.

These guidelines can help increase the effectiveness of a software development program. Whatever the maturity of the current software process, measures of effectiveness and emphasis on continuous improvement can yield significant benefits in increased quality and productivity.

Chapter 18

Laboratory Testing

Compliance in the laboratory is really quite basic. The quality laboratory is responsible for establishing specifications, sampling plans and test procedures for components, in-process materials, and finished products in the developmental and production environments. These plans and procedures must be executed, and the resultant data must be evaluated for conformance to the plans, procedures, and specifications. Each of these activities must be identified in a procedure, and those procedures must be followed. When an auditor reviews the laboratory operation, he or she should observe and inquire about what the laboratory does.

Product testing and laboratory functions can be found in several departmental functions within the medical device firm. The medical device quality control laboratory may be any laboratory that performs physical, chemical, and microbiological tests or performs inspections or tests of components. In-process and finished products are included as part of the laboratory testing function. Laboratories within the research and development are not immune from the requirements of the quality system regulation or cGMP.

The implementation of appropriate, required procedures and the consistent execution of the procedures accomplish compliance with the regulation. Since the Medical Device Quality System Regulation 21 CFR Part 820 does not address laboratory operations, laboratory operations in the devices arena are often evaluated against the pertinent sections of the Finished Pharmaceuticals GMP 21 CFR Part 211. The QSR, 21 CFR Part 820.70 Production and Process Controls includes many of the functions carried out in the quality laboratory.

The laboratory is the center for testing and analyses for the acceptance or rejection of components, in-process materials, and finished products. The biological laboratory normally is responsible for monitoring the production environment for the control of contamination and is often the responsible group for sterilization process validation. Laboratory personnel are required to have the education, training, and experience, or any combination thereof, to enable each person to perform their assigned functions.

The auditor makes a judgment by determining if there are approved procedures for each activity that the procedures are adequate, the procedures are being followed, and if what the laboratory does is adequate.

Laboratory procedures should include the following elements:

- Define the purpose and scope of the procedure.

- List the responsibilities of those performing the procedure.

- List the materials and equipment necessary to perform the procedure.

- Provide a detailed description of the steps to be performed.

- Indicate where and how required data are to be recorded.

- Evaluate data against established specifications.

- Provide directions for actions to be taken when a problem is identified with the performance of the procedure.

The quality control testing laboratory should have the necessary procedures that describe all testing and operational activities. The procedures fall into the following general categories:

- Management systems

- Testing and operating procedures

- Data accountability

- Methods validation

- Personnel training

- Equipment

- Facilities

- Documentation

DEFINITIONS

bioburden—population of viable microorganisms on a given component, package, and finished device after manufacturing.

presterilization count—population of viable microorganisms on a product or package prior to sterilization.

recovery efficiency—measure of the ability of a specific technique to remove and culture microorganisms from a test article.

APPLICABLE STANDARDS FOR LABORATORY TESTING

- United States Pharmacopoeia/National Formulary (USP/NF)

- ISO 11737-1 Sterilization of Medical Devices—Microbiological Methods—Part 1: Estimation of Population of Microorganisms on Products

- Guideline of the Limulus Amebocyte Lysate (LAL) Test As an End-Product Endotoxin Test for Human and Animal Parenteral Drugs, Biological Products, and Medical Devices, 1987

MANAGEMENT SYSTEMS

The regulations require accountability for quality management. In the laboratory, for example, the manager or supervisors are held accountable for the review of analytical raw data, and for the work performed and the review of the analysts' data. The management system shall provide for the notification of the manager or supervisor when out of specification (OOS) test results are found. Procedures for the management system should include the following:

- Handling OOS test results

- Notification of management of OOS results

- Investigation of OOS results and deviations

- Treatment of outliner results

- Procedures for the auditing and approval of contract testing laboratories

OPERATING AND TESTING PROCEDURES

Operating procedures that describe good laboratory practices assure that testing is performed accurately and according to approved test methods. The operating procedures provide control and describe sampling and sampling plans and provide accountability of articles tested in the laboratory. Operating procedures should provide control of the following:

- Personnel attire

- Purchase, receipt, storage, labeling, and control of test samples

  - Name of material

  - Lot/batch number

  - Container from which the sample was taken

  - Date/time of sampling

  - Name of sampler

- Purchase, receipt, storage, labeling, and control of chemicals, culture media, and reagents

- Purchase, receipt, storage, labeling, and control of laboratory reference standards, gauges, and analytical chromatography columns

- Expiration dating of standards and reagents

- Laboratory and glassware cleaning

Testing and inspection procedures describe critical equipment, materials, and steps to be used to determine conformance to specifications of the articles and systems being tested. Testing and inspection procedures should provide control of the following.

Receiving Inspection

- Quality inspection plans and accept/reject specifications for components and materials

- Inspection techniques and measurement equipment/instruments

BIOLOGICAL TESTING

The biological laboratory is normally the group that performs environmental monitoring programs of critical systems. The standards and procedures used for environmental monitoring program activities are described in chapter 12. The lab will in most cases perform product release or sterilization validation biological indicator testing if ethylene oxide, steam, or dry-heat processes are used for sterilization. The standards and procedures used for sterilization validation activities are described in chapter 13.

- Challenge of microbiological test media (growth promotion)

- Preparation, storage, and control of microbiological test media

- Bacterial endotoxin test procedures

- Bioburden testing (products and packaging)

- Environmental monitoring programs of facilities systems (production environments, HVAC, water systems, compressed air systems)

- Biological indicator, BI sterility testing

- Product sterility testing associated with radiation sterilization validations and dose audits

ANALYTICAL TESTING

In medical device products, chemical analyses are not routinely utilized, but may be limited to UV spectrophotometric and FTIR analysis for the identification of component materials. For in vitro diagnostics, more involved chemical analyses are often the case. Testing procedures should provide control of the following:

- Preparation of standards

- Expiration dating of standards

- Preparation, storage, and control of chromatographic mobile phases

- Procedures are to contain specifications or acceptable limits

Methods Validation

Validation of biological and chemical analytical test methods is an essential element of the laboratory management system. It is critical that test methods be validated to determine the appropriateness and validity of the analyses being performed. The validation of test methods is coupled with the validation of critical equipment used to perform the test.

Sterility Testing

In the case of medical devices, product sterility tests are performed primarily in association with the validation of the sterilization process and are not performed as a test for product release. The sterility tests of biological indicators, those that are used to monitor the sterilization process, are tested for product/process release.

The validations of sterility tests are described in the USP/NF and the specific sterilization standard utilized for process validation.

Bioburden Testing

A sterile product item is one that is free of viable microorganisms. The international standards for sterilization of healthcare products require, when it is necessary to supply a sterile product item, that adventitious microbiological contamination of a healthcare product from all sources is minimized by all practical means. Products that are produced under standard manufacturing conditions may have microorganisms on them, although in low numbers. Such items are nonsterile and the purpose of the sterilization process is to inactivate the microbiological contaminants and thereby transform the nonsterile items into sterile ones.

The validations of procedures for the estimation of microbiological populations are outlined in ISO 11737-1 Sterilization of Medical Devices—Microbiological Methods—Part 1: Estimation of Population of Microorganisms on Products. The critical element is that a recovery factor be established for the methods utilized.

Bacterial Endotoxin Testing

Medical devices that are required to be pyrogen-free are tested by an assay for bacterial endotoxins. The test is the limulus amebocyte lysate (LAL) test and may utilize gel clot, kinetic-turbidimetric, or chromogenic methods. Compendial procedures are outlined in the USP and validation procedures are listed in the FDA Guideline of the Limulus Amebocyte Lysate Test as an end-product endotoxin test for human and animal parenteral drugs, biological products, and medical devices.

Environmental Testing

Monitoring of the manufacturing environments is normally an activity performed by the biological laboratory. The critical element of environmental and facilities/utilities monitoring (HVAC/water systems) is that specifications (alert/action-levels/limits) be established and these specifications be established based upon a statistical application. Water system specifications can be found in the USP. Environmental monitoring and control are addressed in chapter 12.

Analytical Testing

GMPs require that methods be validated. Validation of analytical methods basically means that documentation exists to prove that a method used is accurate, sensitive, and specific and will reproducibly yield reliable results. Validation is required for non-compendial methods (those not codified in the USP or other internationally accepted standard methods). The following elements of analytical methods validation are addressed in the USP:

- Accuracy
- Precision
- Linearity
- Specificity
- Range
- Limit of detection
- Limit of quantitation
- Ruggedness and robustness

Equipment

Each piece of critical equipment in the laboratory is to have a unique identification. Procedures are to be established for the operation and maintenance are to be written and approved.

Validation

In the laboratory each piece of critical equipment requires validation or qualification. Procedure or protocols are to be written and approved that list the criteria by which validation and qualifications are performed. The procedures or protocols should include installation qualification (IQ), operational qualification (OQ), and performance qualification (PQ). The procedures or protocols are applicable to test and calibration instrumentation, inspection tools (apparatus and gages), incubators/ovens, refrigerators, autoclaves, and so on. Basically, any instrument that measures a condition of a test.

Calibration

In the laboratory, each piece of critical equipment requires calibration. Each item requiring calibration is to be covered by a procedure and be recalibrated at a time period described in the calibration program. One of the first keys to evaluate in a laboratory regarding calibration is the status of each instrument. Elements of the calibration include:

- A procedure describing the calibration steps
- Established intervals and tolerance limits
- Standards are identified and traceable
- Documentation of each calibration
- Procedures to follow when instruments fail calibration

Personnel Training

The most critical element in the laboratory is an effective training program. Analysts are to be trained in the specific methods each perform, and that training is to be conducted and documented by qualified individuals. Training is to occur continuously or on an ongoing basis. A key indicator of GMP compliance in the laboratory is the training process used when new procedures are introduced or existing procedures are revised.

Data Accountability

In the arena of raw data, GMP requires a complete record of all data secured in the course of each test, including all graphs, charts, and spectra from laboratory instrumentation, and a record of all calculations performed in connection with the test, including units of measure, conversion factors, and equivalency factors. Procedures in the laboratory should include at least the following:

- Handling of raw laboratory data
- Identification of instrument printouts
- Averaging results, rounding, and significant figures
- Second-party review of laboratory data
- Entry of data into LIMS (if applicable)
- Changing data in LIMS (if applicable)

Facilities

The laboratory facilities, like the facilities of the manufacturing areas, are to be in a state of control. This is applicable to HVAC, water, and equipment as well. Procedures are to be in place to demonstrate control. Procedures governing the laboratory consist of the following:

- Safety and handling of hazardous materials, including the decontamination of biological wastes
- Cleaning and sanitization of the work surfaces and laboratory equipment
- Proper identification of labeling, equipment, and instrumentation

Documentation

GMP requires that laboratory procedures shall be written, adequate to describe the activity, and all operations must conform to these procedures. In most laboratories several types of procedures exist. Each document must be controlled. That is, a mechanism must exist in which all documents are approved before they become official, and a controlled means for making document changes must exist. Without proper controls one can never be sure that the method and procedures in use are correct. Procedures for documentation in the laboratory should address the following topics:

- Good documentation practices
- Use of laboratory notebooks and data sheets

- Control of laboratory notebooks and data sheets
- Forms control
- Handling deviations to sampling and test procedures
- Documenting and handling of OOS results
- Preparation of protocols and reports

Part III
International Standards and Guidance

Chapter 19
International Quality System Guidance

This chapter specifically deals with standards and other guidance documents. No discussion of ISO 9000:1994 or ISO 9000:2000 is included, as there are a number of available texts and references that specifically discuss those topics.

OVERVIEW OF EUROPEAN HARMONIZED STANDARDS

Article 5 of the Active Implantable Medical Devices Directive (AIMD), Medical Device Directive (MDD), and In Vitro Diagnostic Device Directive (IVDD) state that the European Economic Area (EEA) countries must presume a device complies with the essential requirements if the device is in conformity with the relevant harmonized EN standard(s).The harmonized standards are published in a listing in the *Official Journal of the European Communities.*

DISCUSSION

Since the medical device directives lay down the essential requirements in very general terms, standards can be important guides to the manufacturer. Standards interpret the safety objectives and also provide the technical route to compliance.

While compliance with the essential requirements of directives is mandatory, the use of harmonized standards is voluntary. However, the following order of standards is most likely to assure compliance.

HARMONIZED STANDARDS

The most direct route to compliance through standards is the use of harmonized standards. A manufacturer who uses harmonized standards in the design and production of devices is presumed in conformity with the essential requirements. The use of harmonized standards is the most direct route to compliance with any of the medical device directives.

INTERNATIONAL STANDARDS

Where no harmonized standards exist, manufacturers may use standards that are issued from international standards developing organizations such as the ISO and IEC.

NATIONAL STANDARDS

The third-best choice is the use of European national standards, to be used when no harmonized standards or international standards exist. Also, other sources such as AAMI, ASTM, and the FDA may be considered.

The principle of applying standards, therefore, is the following:

Harmonized standards that have been developed specifically to deal with the essential requirements of the medical device directives provide an assumption of conformity. In their absence, the manufacturer is entitled to comply with any appropriate specifications that may demonstrate conformity with the essential requirements. However, the manufacturer must bear the burden of proving that the use of specifications or standards other than harmonized standards supports the product meeting the essential requirements.

A manufacturer may decide not to use an existing harmonized standard, but if this is done the burden is on the manufacturer to show the standards or specifications used fulfill the same requirements. This approach is not recommended unless there are mitigating circumstances.

Chapter 20
The EU Medical Device Directives

The EU medical device directives:

- Active Implantable Medical Devices Directive 90/385 EEC (AIMD)
- Medical Device Directive 93/42 EEC (MDD)
- In Vitro Diagnostic Directive 79/98 EC (IVDD)

Medical devices and in vitro diagnostic products that are to be placed on the market in the EEA are required to bear a CE marking. The requirements for this are defined in three European directives. The directives break the medical device market into three areas for regulatory purposes:

- Active implantable medical devices (AIMD)
- Medical devices (MDD)
- In vitro diagnostic devices (IVDD)

The three directives need to be considered as a set since the AIMD was amended by the MDD and the IVDD amended the MDD. The AIMD and MDD are mandatory, and any device the falls under them must have a CE marking in order to be placed on the market in the EEA.

DEFINITIONS

Article 1 of the AIMD, MDD, IVDD define some key terms. These are listed next and referred to in later sections. The following definitions are as amended by the IVDD.

medical device—any instrument, apparatus, appliance, material, or other article, whether used alone or in combination, including the software necessary for its proper application, intended by the manufacturer to be used for human beings for the purpose of:

- Diagnosis, prevention, monitoring, treatment, or alleviation of disease
- Diagnosis, monitoring, treatment, alleviation, or compensation for an injury or handicap

- Investigation, replacement or modification of the anatomy or of a physiological process

- Control of conception

and that does not achieve its principal intended action in or on the human body by pharmacological, immunological, or metabolic means, but which may be assisted in its function by such means.

accessory—an article that, while not being a device, is intended specifically by its manufacturer to be used together with a device to enable it to be used in accordance with the use of the device intended by the manufacturer of the device.

active medical device—any medical device relying for its functioning on a source of electrical energy or any source of power other than that directly generated by the human body or gravity.

active implantable medical device—any active medical device that is intended to be totally or partially introduced, surgically or medically, into the human body or by medical intervention into a natural orifice, and that is intended to remain after the procedure.

in vitro diagnostic medical device—any medical device that is a reagent, reagent product, calibrator, control material, kit, instrument, apparatus, equipment, or system, whether used alone or in combination, intended by the manufacturer to be used in vitro for the examination of specimens, including blood and tissue donations, derived from the human body, solely or principally for the purpose of providing information: 1) concerning a physiological or pathological state; 2) concerning a congenital abnormality; 3) to determine the safety and compatibility with potential recipients; or 4) to monitor therapeutic measures.

Specimen receptacles are considered to be in vitro diagnostic medical devices. Specimen receptacles are those devices, whether vacuum-type or not, specifically intended by their manufacturers for the primary containment and preservation of specimens derived from the human body for the purpose of in vitro diagnostic examination.

Products for general laboratory use are not in vitro diagnostic medical devices unless such products, in view of their characteristics, are specifically intended by their manufacturer to be used for in vitro diagnostic examination.

IVD accessory—an article that, while not being an in vitro diagnostic medical device, is intended specifically by its manufacturer to be used together with a device to enable that device to be used in accordance with its intended purpose.

Invasive sampling devices or those that are directly applied to the human body for the purpose of obtaining a specimen within the meaning of Directive 93/42/EEC shall not be considered to be accessories to in vitro diagnostic medical devices.

device for self-testing—any device intended by the manufacturer to be able to be used by lay persons in a home environment.

manufacturer—the natural or legal person with responsibility for the design, manufacture, packaging, and labeling of a device before it is placed on the market under his own name, regardless of whether these operations are carried out by that person or on his or her behalf by a third party. The obligations of this directive to be met by manufacturers also apply to the natural or legal person who assembles, packages, processes, fully refurbishes, and/or labels one or more ready-made products and/or assigns to them their intended purpose as devices with a view to their being placed on the market under his or her own name. This subparagraph does not apply to the person who, while not a manufacturer within the meaning of the first subparagraph, assembles or adapts devices already on the market to their intended purpose for an individual patient.

authorized representative—any natural or legal person established in the community who, explicitly designated by the manufacturer, acts and may be addressed by authorities and bodies in the community instead of the manufacturer with regard to the latter's obligations under this directive.

PURPOSE OF THE MEDICAL DEVICE DIRECTIVES

The purpose of the EU medical device directives is to harmonize the regulations and administrative provisions among the member states of the EEA and ensure the safety, health, protection, and performance characteristics of medical devices and in vitro diagnostic devices.

The format of the directives consists of a number of articles that cover definitions, scope, free movement of CE marked devices, standards, conformity assessment, and reporting of device incidents. These are followed by a number of annexes, which cover the essential requirements for product safety and performance, conformity assessment procedures, and classification criteria.

Before a manufacturer can place the CE marking on a medical device and legally sell to, or within the EEA, it must be in compliance with the applicable directive.

REQUIREMENTS FOR COMPLIANCE

The following items are required for compliance with the directives:

- Determination whether the product has to comply with one of the directives
- Classification of devices
- Conformity assessment routes
- Compliance with the essential requirements
- Harmonized standards
- Risk analysis
- Technical file/design dossier
- Authorized representative
- Device incident reporting/the vigilance system
- CE marking
- Declaration of conformity

DETERMINING WHETHER THE PRODUCT HAS TO COMPLY WITH THE MEDICAL DEVICE DIRECTIVES

Regulatory requirements: AIMD, MDD and IVDD: The definition of an active implantable medical device, a medical device, or an in vitro diagnostic device is defined in article 1 of each directive. The definitions are provided in the previous section. The definitions have been amended by the IVDD so they should be referred to even if dealing with a medical device and not an IVD. If a product meets the criteria as defined in article 1 of any of the directives then the manufacturer must comply with the appropriate directive. A device is only governed by one of the directives.

Accessories to an AIMD, MDD, or IVDD device are treated as the same type of device. The only exception is accessories to IVD products that are used for invasive sampling. These are treated as a medical device.

DISCUSSION

The Active Implantable Medical Devices Directive

The active implantable medical devices directive (AIMD) applies to devices and their accessories. The AIMD covers active implantable products such as cardiac pacemakers, defibrillators, infusion pumps, and neurostimulators.

"Active" implies that the function of these devices is dependent upon a source of energy other than gravity or human power. In almost all cases, this is electrical power.

Accessories to AIMD devices are also covered by the AIMD. Accessories and software, such as external pacemaker programming devices, are governed by the AIMD even though they are not directly implanted.

Medical Device Directive

The medical device directive (MDD) applies to medical devices and their accessories. The MDD covers nonactive implantable products such as heart valves and orthopedic implants, surgically invasive devices such as catheters and surgical instruments, and noninvasive devices such as extracorporeal tubing and kidney dialysis modules. The MDD also covers active devices such as ventilators, patient monitors, and electrosurgical equipment,

A medical device is defined in the MDD article 1 and was listed previously. In addition, the MDD covers accessories and software that are used with a medical device. Examples include the software used to control or program radiation treatment. The software, if provided separately, has the same classification as the device with which it is used.

In Vitro Diagnostic Directive

The in vitro diagnostic directive (IVDD) applies to in vitro medical devices and their accessories. The IVDD covers products such as blood glucose devices used for self-testing, blood analysis test equipment and reagents, home pregnancy test kits, and blood collection tubes.

The IVDD also covers the calibration kits and products used to calibrate IVD test equipment. As mentioned previously, if a sample collection device is invasive, such as a blood lancet or invasive swab, then that device is covered under the MDD.

CLASSIFICATION OF MEDICAL DEVICES

The three directives follow different approaches in terms of classifying or categorizing devices. The classification/categorization is important as it determines the requirements for conformity assessment for the device.

AIMD

There are no classifications or categories of devices within the AIMD.

MDD

Devices are classified according to the requirements of the MDD article 9 and the rules in Annex IX.

IVDD

The IVDD provides a list of specific IVD devices in Annex II, which is divided into list A and B. In addition, devices for self-testing are also treated as a separate category for conformity assessment.

DISCUSSION

AIMD

All devices covered by the AIMD are treated the same; there are no classes or categories of devices in the AIMD. The conformity assessment requirements apply equally to all AIMD devices.

MDD

Devices are classified into one of four classifications: class I, class IIa, class IIb, and class III. In addition, there are two additional subsets of class I devices: class I (sterile), class I (with measuring function). Although the last two subsets of class I devices are not a separate classification, they have unique conformity assessment requirements.

MDD Annex IX contains the device classification criteria and rules. Classification depends upon intended use of the device and potential risk of the device. Special attention should be paid to the terms defined in Annex IX, as they have a significant impact on classification.

Devices and their accessories may be classified separately, as individual devices and individual accessories, or together as a system.

IVDD

The IVDD does not follow the same idea of a classification scheme like the MDD. Annex II of the IVDD identifies two lists of specific IVD products that could be considered as classes. Each group in Annex II has specific requirements for conformity assessment. The groups are identified as the list A and list B devices.

In addition, the IVDD has specific requirements for devices used for self-testing by the patient. In essence, there are four classes of IVD devices, Annex II list A, Annex II list B, devices for self-test, and all other IVD devices.

CONFORMITY ASSESSMENT ROUTE

Regulatory requirements: The manufacturer must use a conformity assessment route appropriate to the device. Conformity assessment routes are detailed in the relevant articles and annexes of each directive, and are outlined in the following.

Note: The AIMD uses Arabic numbering and the MDD/IVDD use Roman numerals to number the annexes.

AIMD

Annex 2	Full Quality Assurance System (ISO 9001/ISO 13485)
Annex 3	Type Examination (Product testing)
Annex 4	Type Verification (Batch or unit verification)
Annex 5	Production Quality Assurance System (ISO 9001/ISO 13485)

MDD

Article 11 of the MDD outlines the options for conformity assessment depending on the device classification. The annexes that may be used are:

Annex II	Full Quality Assurance System (ISO 9001/ISO 13485)
Annex III	Type Examination (Product testing)
Annex IV	Type Verification (Batch or unit verification)
Annex V	Production Quality Assurance System (ISO 9001/ISO 13485)
Annex VI	Product Quality Assurance System (ISO 9001/ISO 13485)
Annex VII	Declaration of Conformity (Self-declaration)

IVDD

Article 9 of the IVDD outlies the options for conformity assessment depending on the device category. The annexes that may be used are:

Annex III	Declaration of Conformity (Self-declaration)

Annex IV   Full Quality Assurance System (ISO 9001/ISO 13485)

Annex V   Type Examination (Product testing)

Annex VI   Type Verification (Batch or unit verification)

Annex VII   Production Quality Assurance System (ISO 9001/ISO 13485)

DISCUSSION

AIMD

The acceptable assessment options are:

- Annex II full quality assurance, which consists of an audit by a notified body to the requirements of ISO 9001/ISO 13485 plus submission of the product data in a design dossier for design examination

- Annex III–type examination, which is a full test of the product to the applicable standards and Annex V production quality assurance, which is an audit to ISO 9001/ISO 13485.

- Annex III–type examination combined with Annex IV–type verification, which is a unit-by-unit or batch-by-batch testing of the device

MDD

Conformity assessment options (per MDD Article 11) are dependent upon the device classification:

Class I

Annex VII the manufacturer does self-declaration to the requirements of the MDD; no audit or testing is required

Class I Sterile or with Measurement Function

The manufacturer then uses Annex VII self-declaration combined with an Annex audit to the applicable aspects of sterility or measurement function by the notified body

Annex IV* batch-by-batch-type verification combined with Annex VII self-declaration

Class IIa

Annex II full quality assurance audit to ISO 9001/ISO 13485, but without a design examination

---

*Not applicable to sterile devices

Annex V production quality assurance plus Annex VII self-declaration

Annex IV*–Type verification plus Annex VII self-declaration

Class IIb Devices

Annex II full quality assurance without design examination

Annex III–type examination plus Annex V production quality assurance

Annex III–type examination plus Annex VI* product quality assurance

Annex III–type exam plus Annex IV*–type verification

Class III Devices

Annex II full quality assurance plus design examination

Annex III–type examination plus Annex V production quality assurance

Annex III–type examination plus Annex IV*–type verification

IVDD

Self-Test Devices

Annex III, section 6 the manufacturer submits the device data for a design examination; no audit or testing is required

Annex IV full quality assurance audit to ISO 9001/EN46001 but without a design examination

Annex V production quality assurance plus Annex VII self-declaration

Annex V–type examination plus Annex IV–type verification

Annex II, List A

Annex IV full quality assurance with design examination, plus batch verification per Annex IV, section 6

Annex V–type examination plus Annex VII production quality assurance

Annex II, List B

Annex IV full quality assurance without design examination

Annex V–type examination plus Annex VII production quality assurance

Annex V–type examination plus Annex VI–type verification

All Others

Annex III the manufacturer does self-declaration to the requirements of the IVDD; no audit or testing is required

*Not applicable to sterile devices

COMPLIANCE WITH ESSENTIAL REQUIREMENTS

Regulatory Requirements

All devices that are CE marked must fulfill the essential requirements as defined in Annex I of the AIMD, MDD, or IVDD. Article 3 of the AIMD, MDD, and IVDD require that any device placed on the market with a CE marking complies with the requirements in Annex I.

Discussion

The essential requirements of each directive are contained in Annex I. They describe, in a general way, the safety requirements for the devices covered by the directive, and compliance, where applicable, is mandatory.

The essential requirements in Annex I are divided into general requirements and specific requirements that relate to the design, construction, labeling, and clinical or performance data.

Issues addressed with regard to design and construction include: chemical, physical, and biological properties; infection and microbial contamination; construction and environmental properties; electrical safety; EMC; software validation; and, where applicable, approval of medicinal products or nonviable animal tissue.

All AIMD and MDD devices must also be support by clinical data. Clinical data are either the result of a clinical investigation or a compilation and critical review of available scientific literature.

RISK ANALYSIS

Regulatory Requirement

Each of the three directives requires that the risks versus the benefits to the patient and user are determined. This is defined in several of the parts of Annex I of each directive.

Discussion

The essential requirements of all three directives require the manufacturer to conduct a risk assessment for the device.

The European Committee for Standardization (CEN) has developed the standard EN 1441, which addresses the elements of risk analysis that are related to the devices covered by the AIMD, MDD, and IVDD. This standard has been replaced by EN ISO 14971:2000, which should be used from this point forward.

The directive and the standards all follow a hierarchy of mitigation of risk by:

- Elimination of the hazard by design

- Use of alarms

- Labeling

The manufacturer should have a procedure for performing risk analysis, and a signed risk analysis available for any CE-marked device.

TECHNICAL FILE/DESIGN DOSSIER

Regulatory Requirement

Each conformity assessment annex of the three directives requires the manufacturer to have "technical documentation" for each device. The wording and descriptions vary by directive and annex. The term *technical file* is used to describe the documentation that shows how the device complies with the essential requirements. For devices that require a design examination the technical file is called a *design dossier.*

Discussion

The manufacturer must compile a technical file. This file must contain or point to all the relevant information that is needed to demonstrate that the product meets the essential requirements of the applicable directive. The required contents of the technical file are set out in the selected conformity assessment annex of each directive.

The manufacturer or his authorized representative must make this documentation, including the declaration of conformity, available to the competent authorities of each EEA country for inspection purposes for a period ending at least five years after the last product has been manufactured.

In general, the technical documentation should include:

- Name and address of the manufacturer and European representative

- Product description, including the identification (model name/number) of the product, description of the intended use, accessories for the product (if applicable), integral parts of the sales unit (if applicable), classification of the device and accessories (if applicable), chosen conformity assessment path, and brief product history (including existing regulatory approvals)

- List of harmonized standards followed by the manufacturer and/or the solutions adopted to satisfy the essential requirements

- Overall manufacturing and inspection plans for the product

- Risk analysis

- Clinical data (results of clinical literature review or a clinical investigation)

- Labeling, such as product labels, instructions for use, patient information, and advertising material

- Applicable test data to supporting the fulfillment of the applied harmonized standards and essential requirements, that is, electrical safety data, sterilization validation, software validation, biocompatibility, and so on.

The manufacturer should have a procedure to describe how the technical files are assembled and controlled. A valid file for each device that is CE marked should exist. Also, a procedure should exist to define the collection and preparation of clinical data.

For those devices that require a design dossier, the content is the same, the only difference is the file must be in one physical document so it can be submitted to the notified body.

AUTHORIZED REPRESENTATIVE

Regulatory Requirements

The term *authorized representative* was only fully defined in the IVDD article 1, but the definition applies to all three directives. The requirements are spelled out throughout the directives in both the articles and annexes. The authorized representative's name must appear on the device labeling.

Discussion

The medical device directives require the appointment of an authorized representative for Europe in the event the manufacturer does not have a place of business within the EEA. The manufacturer or authorized representative may also have to register with the competent authority of the member state(s) in which it has a place of business.

The directives require that the authorized representative be listed on the label and/or packaging, or in the instructions.

In addition, the authorized representative must keep the technical file available for review by competent authorities.

DEVICE INCIDENT REPORTING, THE VIGILANCE

Regulatory Requirements

Article 8 of the AIMD, article 10 of the MDD, and article 11 of the IVDD require manufacturers to report incidents involving their devices to the relevant competent authorities. In addition to the requirements defined in the aforementioned articles of each directive, guidance on reporting is provided in the Vigilance Guidance document. This document is MEDDEV 2.12-1 rev 4, April 2001.

Discussion

The manufacturer must institute and keep up to date a systematic procedure to review experience gained from devices in the post-production phase and to implement appropriate means to apply any necessary corrective actions and report device incidents.

Incidents are events that have led to a death or to a serious deterioration in the state of health of a patient, user, or other person. Near incidents are events that might lead to a death or a serious deterioration in health. In assessing the link between the device and the incident or near incident, the manufacturer should take into account:

- The opinion of healthcare professionals, based on valid evidence

- The results of the manufacturer's own preliminary assessment of the incident

- Evidence of previous, similar incidents

- Other evidence held by the manufacturer

The following times are the maximum elapsed times for determining the relevant facts and making an initial report. The time starts from the manufacturer/authorized representative first being informed of the incident, to the relevant competent authority receiving the notification from the manufacturer.

Incidents: 10 days

Near incidents: 30 days

Incidents are reported to the competent authority where the incident occurred. For more details on this the MEDDEV document listed previously should be consulted.

CE MARKING

Regulatory Requirements

The manufacturer is obliged to place the CE marking on the device. Annex IX AIMD (as amended by Directive 93/68/EEC), Annex XII MDD, and Annex XX IVDD instruct the manufacturer on the placing of the CE marking. Article 12 of the AIMD, article 17 of the MDD, and article 16 of the IVDD also define requirements for placement of the CE marking.

Discussion

The CE marking must be either on the device or its primary package, the shipping/ sales package, and the instructions for use. Reusable devices must have the CE marking on the device. The CE marking must appear as defined in the annexes listed previously. It must be at least 5 mm high.

The CE marking in most cases must also include the number of the notified body used. The only exceptions are for class 1 MDD devices that are nonsterile and do not have a measuring function. IVDD devices that are in the self-declaration category also do not have a notified body number attached.

DECLARATION OF CONFORMITY

Regulatory Requirements

Each conformity assessment annex as listed previously requires that the manufacturer issue a declaration of conformity prior to shipping products with a CE marking.

Discussion

The manufacturer must draw up a declaration of conformity prior to CE-marking a device and keep a copy available.

The declaration of conformity must usually contain the following elements:

- Manufacturer: name and address
- European representative: name and address
- Product: name, type and/or model
- Classification: class, rule according to Annex IX of the MDD

- Standards applied: list of (harmonized) standards for which documented evidence for compliance can be provided

- Notified body: name, address and identification number
  EC Certificate(s): EC certificate(s) number(s)

- Start of CE marking: date, lot number or serial number of first CE marking

- Place, date of issue: city, date

- Signature

Chapter 21

International Auditing Guidelines

GHTF AUDITING GUIDELINES

GHTF SG4 (99) 28, *Guidelines for Regulatory Auditing of Quality Systems of Medical Device Manufacturers—Part 1: General Requirements,* was developed by Study Group 4 of the Global Harmonization Task Force (GHTF). Although auditing organizations are the target audience for this document, it is a useful guidance for medical device manufactures and auditors of these establishments. The following chapter outlines the requirements of the GHTF guidance document.

Audit Objectives

Quality audits are designed to determine if the quality system:

- Complies with regulatory and recognized quality standard requirements
- Meets customers' contractual requirements
- Achieves its objectives and conforms to internal requirements
- Is effectively implemented

Audits are also used to evaluate whether prior corrective actions have been adequately and effectively implemented.

Definitions

The following definitions are provided in GHTF SG4 (99) 28, *Guidelines for Regulatory Auditing of Quality Systems of Medical Device Manufacturers—Part 1: General Requirements,* GHTF SG4 (00) 3, *Training Requirements for Auditors,* and GHTF SG4 (99) 14, *Audit Language Requirements.*

audit—a systematic and independent examination to determine whether quality activities and related results comply with planned arrangements and whether these arrangements are implemented effectively and are suitable to achieve objectives.

auditee—any organization whose quality systems are to be audited for compliance with the relevant medical device regulatory requirements.

audit language—the language(s) routinely used for the communication or exchange of information between auditee's personnel and auditors.

auditing organization—a body designated, on the basis of specific regulations, to carry out audits according to assigned tasks.

auditor—a person with relevant qualifications and competence to perform audits or specified parts of such audits and who belongs to, or is authorized by, the auditing organization.

lead auditor—an auditor designated to manage an audit (also known as an audit team leader).

manufacturer—the legal entity subject by regulation to quality system requirements.

nonconformity—the nonfulfillment of specified requirements within the planned arrangements. Other terms may be used to mean the same as nonconformity (for example, noncompliance, deficiency).

objective evidence—verifiable information or records pertaining to the quality of an item or service or to the existence and implementation of a quality system element, which is based on visual observation, measurement, or test.

quality audit observation—statement of fact made during a quality audit and substantiated by objective evidence.

quality system—the organizational structure, responsibilities, procedures, processes, and resources for implementing quality management.

regulatory requirements—any part of a law, ordinance, decree, or other regulation that applies to quality systems of medical device manufacturers. Guidelines, notes, draft documents, or the like should not be used as regulatory documents and are not to be construed as such unless formally promulgated.

training elements—topics within a training program that describe the content for addressing a particular training need.

Types of Audits

Audits can be classified into four categories: initial audit, surveillance audit, special audit, and unannounced audit.

During an initial audit, all elements of the quality system will be audited. A surveillance audit is conducted after the initial audit and can include all or some quality system elements. If the auditing organization performs partial surveillance audits, all elements of the quality system should be reviewed within a maximum period of five years.

The time between surveillance audits will depend on the:

- Risk associated with the medical devices

- Number of quality system elements examined

- Nature of the quality system elements examined

- Scope and results of the previous audits

- Available post-market surveillance data

Special audits are performed when a possible significant deficiency in the quality system is indicated or the auditing body becomes aware of significant safety-related information. They can also occur if there are significant changes to the quality system that could affect the state of compliance. Unannounced audits are not typical, but may be conducted if the auditing organization has significant compliance concerns.

GENERAL AUDITING PRINCIPLES

Independence

The audit process should ensure objectivity and impartiality. The auditing organization and its auditors should perform their duties in an independent and objective manner and avoid any potential conflict of interest. They should not audit their own work or areas in which they are directly involved (financially or professionally). They must be unbiased and independent of the area being audited in order to permit objective completion of the audit. Independence should be regularly assessed. Factors to consider include personal relationships, financial interests, and prior job assignments and responsibilities.

Audit Objectives and Scope

During the planning stages of the audit, the auditing organization, the auditor, or the audit team must define and document the audit objectives and audit scope. Defining the objectives and scope enables efficient use of time and resources. The objectives define what is to be accomplished. The scope establishes boundaries and identifies what is to be examined. The following should be considered when establishing the audit scope:

- Medical devices manufactured

- Quality system requirements

- Type of audit (initial, surveillance, or special)

- Physical location of activities and documentation

If applicable and appropriate, these should be provided to the auditee for review and approval. It is feasible that, during the course of the audit, the objectives and/or scope may change based on audit observations and nonconformances noted.

Roles, Responsibilities, and Authorities

The roles, responsibility, authority, and accountability of all organizations and individuals involved with the audit process should be appropriately identified, defined, and documented. This includes the auditing organization, the lead auditor, the auditor(s), the auditee, and the manufacturer (if different from the auditee). This can be done as part of the audit planning process or a "generic" outline can be part of the auditing organization's SOPs.

Areas to consider for the auditing organization include:

- Assessment of compliance with relevant standards, regulations, and guidelines
- Code of ethics
- Management of the audit process
- Functions to be audited
- Scope or any limitations of scope
- Auditee requirements, rights, and expectations
- Key performance indicators and other measures of performance
- Organizational structure
- Right of access to information, personnel, locations, and systems relevant to the performance of audits
- Risk assessment
- Training, selecting, and supervising auditors
- Methods to ensure consistency in the interpretation of the regulatory requirements
- Audit language
- Completion dates
- Deliverables and method of safeguarding confidentiality
- Intended recipients of deliverables
- Budgets/fees if applicable

An auditor's job is to:

- Evaluate the quality system
- Carry out assigned audit tasks
- Comply with audit requirements
- Cooperate with the lead auditor
- Respect all confidentiality requirements
- Collect evidence about the quality system
- Document audit observations and conclusions
- Safeguard audit documents, records, and reports

- Determine whether quality policy is being applied
- Find out if the quality objectives are being achieved
- See whether quality procedures are being followed
- Verify that effective corrective actions have been implemented
- Help the manufacturer understand the regulatory requirements
- Assist the lead auditor in preparing the audit report

In addition to the aforementioned responsibilities, the lead audit must also:

- Manage the audit
- Identify and assign audit tasks
- Assist in selecting audit team members
- Orient the audit team
- Prepare the audit plan
- Clarify quality audit requirements
- Communicate audit requirements
- Prepare audit forms and checklists
- Preview quality system documents, if appropriate
- Report nonconformities as soon as possible
- Interact with auditee's management
- Present findings at the closing meeting
- Prepare and submit audit reports in a timely manner

The responsibilities of the manufacturer are:

- Define the purpose and scope of the audit
- Determine which standards should be used to evaluate compliance
- Describe the nature, purpose, and scope of the audit to relevant employees
- Appoint responsible employees to accompany and assist the audit team
- Ensure cooperation with the audit team
- Provide the necessary resources for the audit team
- Allow auditors to examine all documents, records, and facilities
- Receive and review the audit report
- Inform the auditing organization of significant quality system changes
- Determine necessary corrective actions to be taken and implement

Resources

In order to ensure reliable audit results and conclusions, there must be adequate resources (competent staff, financial support, time, technical information, external expertise, and so on) dedicated to the audit process and associated auditing activities.

Competence of the Audit Team

A lead auditor, with the competence to plan and manage an audit, as well as direct team members, must be included on the audit team. If the team consists of only one auditor, then this individual will be the lead.

The audit team must possess the necessary professional and technical competence, as a whole, to cover the scope of the audit. The team should be competent with respect to understanding:

- Applicable regulatory, statutory, and safety requirements

- Appropriate device technologies and processes

- Auditing of medical device manufacturers' quality systems

Other areas to consider in assessing competence include professional qualifications, education, skills, training, experience, and personal attributes. If the necessary technical competence is not present within the audit team, additional experts in processes and technology relevant to the scope of the audit may be included or team members may be provided specialized training.

Records to demonstrate the competence of auditors must be maintained by the auditing organization.

Consistency of Procedures

In order to ensure consistency of audits, the audit process, including the responsibilities and requirements for managing, planning, and conducting audits; reporting results; and maintaining records should be defined and documented. These procedures must address applicable regulatory and quality requirements.

Adequacy of Audit Documentation

The auditor or audit team needs to obtain documented evidence to achieve the audit objectives effectively. Documentation associated with each audit should include any information that is required by government regulations or regulatory authorities. Procedures should be in place to ensure adequate retention of the documentation or a time sufficient to satisfy legal, professional, and organizational requirements.

Documentation maintained may include a record of the:

- Audit scope and objectives

- Audit program

- Audit process

- Audit evidence gathered

- Audit findings, conclusions, and recommendations
- Any report issued

Confidentiality, Due Professional Care, and Code of Ethics

The audit process should maintain the confidentiality of information obtained during the course of the audit, unless disclosure is allowed by the auditee or required by legal authority. Information obtained during the audit process should not be used for personal benefit.

Due professional care, good judgment, and observance of applicable auditing standards and requirements should extend to every aspect of the audit and the audit management process.

Quality System

Auditing organizations should implement and maintain a quality system to ensure that the audits conducted are of the highest quality and to facilitate continuous improvement.

Audit Process

While the audit process has been described in many manners by many experts, it has traditionally been divided into four or five phases or stages. The GHTF [GHTF SG4 (99) 28] also details a five-stage approach, as shown in Figure 21.1.

Stage 1: Audit Preparation

The GHTF guidance subdivides this stage into the following tasks: notification, preview of quality system description, site visit audit plan, audit team assignments, and working documents. Portions of the audit preparation process, such as notification and preview of quality system description, are not applicable to those situations where unannounced audits are deemed necessary by the auditing organization.

Unless regulatory requirements mandate otherwise, the auditee should be notified in advance that an audit is to be conducted. Before the on-site examination, the lead auditor should conduct a desk audit of the quality system to determine if the implemented controls meet the regulatory requirements. This can be accomplished by reviewing the quality manual and, if applicable, top-level SOPs. Although this preview is done during the preparation stages, it is actually part of audit execution. If it becomes obvious during the review that the documented system is inadequate, the on-site audit should be suspended until necessary corrective actions are made.

The lead auditor must also develop an audit plan. Where permitted by regulations, the documented plan should be submitted to the manufacturer for approval before the site visit. The audit plan should:

- Define the objectives and scope of the audit.
- Identify the manufacturer's management team having direct responsibility for the audit scope and purpose.

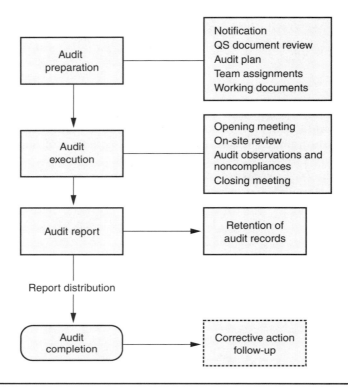

Figure 21.1 Audit process.

- Record the documents that will be audited.
- Identify the applicable audit standards and other reference documents to be utilized.
- Identify the quality elements that will be audited.
- Identify the lead auditor and other team members.
- Specify the language of the audit.
- Specify when and where the audit will be conducted.
- Identify the organizational units and areas that will be audited.
- Define the time and duration for each major audit activity.
- Schedule meetings to be held with the manufacturer's management.
- Identify who will get the final audit report and when.

It is important to note that audit plans are subject to change. During the course of the audit, the objectives and/or scope may change, or become unattainable, based on audit observations and nonconformances noted. The manufacturer must be notified of any changes.

It is the lead auditor's responsibility to assign specific tasks to audit team members. These tasks should be assigned according to the participant's qualifications and expertise.

Working documents are required when performing an audit to international auditing guidelines. Again, it is the lead auditor's responsibility to prepare the working documents; team members should assist as appropriate. Examples of working documents include checklists (to evaluate the system elements against regulatory requirements) and forms (to record observations and collect supporting evidence).

Stage 2: Audit Execution

The audit execution stage should start with an opening meeting with the manufacturer's senior management. The purpose of this meeting is to:

- Introduce the audit team

- Restate, and clarify if necessary, the audit scope, objectives, plan, and schedule

- Review the methods and procedures to be used during the audit

- Confirm that the necessary resources and facilities to support the audit process are available

- Establish communication links

During the on-site assessment, applicable elements of the quality system are evaluated. Objective evidence is collected by:

- Interviewing and questioning personnel

- Reviewing records and documents

- Visually observing activities and conditions

Wherever possible, evidence collected through personnel interviews should be confirmed by other means. Documents or copies of records collected, or any photographs taken, should be noted by the auditors and acknowledged by the auditee. Sampling of records and documents should be appropriate to the risks associated with the device, the complexity of manufacturing technologies, and available post-market surveillance data.

Upon evaluation of the objective evidence collected, auditors must document their quality audit observations (a statement of fact made during a quality audit and substantiated by objective evidence). Nonconformities (nonfulfillment of specified requirements within the planned arrangements), and quality audit observations that have the potential to become nonconformities, should be reviewed with the manufacturer as they are noted.

Nonconformities must be supported by the evidence collected and identify the requirements that have been violated. One or more major nonconformities will indicate that the manufacturer does not comply with the regulatory requirements.

The following are examples of quality audit observations that may be considered nonconformities:

- Lack of or failure to implement a quality system requirement

- Product safety or performance is/may be compromised

- Large number of minor nonconformances against a quality system requirement

- Failure to implement appropriate corrective and preventive actions

- Repeat observations

A closing meeting is held at the completion of the on-site evaluation. The purpose of this meeting is for the lead auditor to discuss quality audit observations, nonconformances, severity of the nonconformances, and overall conclusions with the manufacturer's senior management, and those individuals responsible for the areas audited, before a final report is prepared. The audit team presents a list of audit observations and nonconformities to the management team at this time. The management provides a date to the auditing organization for submission of a corrective action plan to address the nonconformities.

Stage 3: Audit Report

The audit report is the method of formally communicating the audit scope and objectives, the audit plan, the standards and methodology utilized, the objective evidence collected, and the quality audit observations, nonconformities, conclusions, and recommendations. The audit findings and conclusions should be consistent, accurate, and supported by the evidence gathered throughout the audit process.

The lead auditor is responsible for preparing, dating, signing, and submitting the audit report to the manufacturer. Nonconformities identified in the audit report should be specific in nature and include the following:

- Requirements of the internal or external standard

- Severity with respect to the requirements

- Required date for submission of corrective action plans

The audit plan identifies who is to receive the final report and when. If the report cannot be made available to the manufacturer within this period, the auditing organization must notify the manufacturer, provide the reasons for the delay, and establish a new issue date.

Stage 4: Retention of Audit Records

The auditing organization is responsible for retaining all auditing documents for the period of time specified by the applicable regulatory requirements.

Stage 5: Audit Completion

The audit is considered complete upon transmittal of the audit report to the manufacturer.

Corrective Action Follow-Up

The manufacturer is expected to take actions to correct identified nonconformities. The auditing organization and the manufacturer should agree upon a plan for completing necessary corrective actions, and if required, re-audits to verify that corrective actions were taken. Periodic reports may also be requested by the auditing organization to determine the status of the necessary corrective actions.

Appendix A

Biomedical Auditor Certification (CBA) Body of Knowledge

I. Auditing Fundamentals [15 Questions]

    A. *Purpose & types of audits*
Differentiate various audit types (such as product, process, system, management, compliance, first-party, second-party, third-party, internal, external, desk, department, and function) and examine how audits are used to assess organizational effectiveness, system efficiency, process effectiveness, business performance, risk management, and conformance to requirements. (Analyze)

    B. *Roles and responsibilities during an audit*

        1. *Participants and their roles and responsibilities*
Explain the functions and responsibilities of various audit participants, including audit team members, lead auditor, client, auditee, etc. (Apply)

        2. *Ethical, legal, and professional issues*
Identify and apply factors of ethical and professional conduct, concepts of due diligence/due care with respect to confidentiality, conflict of interest, credibility, independence, objectivity, and qualifications. Identify legal and financial ramifications of improper auditor actions, such as carelessness, negligence, and discovery of illegal activities or unsafe conditions. Anticipate the effect that certain audit results can have on an auditee's regulatory and civil liability. (Apply)

II. Auditing & Inspection Processes [30 Questions]

    A. *Audit preparation & planning*

        1. *Elements of the audit planning process*
Determine and implement steps in audit preparation and planning, such as verifying audit authority, establishing the purpose, scope, and type of audit, the requirements to audit against, and the resources necessary, including the size and number of audit teams. (Evaluate)

2. *Auditor selection*
   Identify and examine various auditor selection criteria, such as education, experience, industry background, and subject-matter expertise, and the characteristics that make auditors effective, such as interpersonal skills, problem-solving skills, attention to detail, cultural sensitivity, ability to work independently and in a group or on a team. (Analyze)

3. *Audit-related documentation*
   Identify sources of pre-audit information and examine audit-related documentation, such as reference materials and prior audits. (Analyze)

4. *Auditing tools*
   Select, prepare, and use checklists, log sheets, sampling plans, and procedural guidelines in various audit situations. (Analyze)

5. *Auditing strategies*
   Identify and use various tactical methods for conducting an audit, such as forward and backward tracing and discovery. (Apply)

6. *Logistics*
   Identify and organize various audit-related logistics, such as travel, security considerations, and escorts. (Apply)

B. *Audit performance*

1. *Opening meeting*
   Describe the purpose and scope of an opening meeting, and the necessary elements for conducting such a meeting. (Apply)

2. *Data collection and analysis*
   Select and apply various data collection methods, such as observing work activities, taking physical measurements, examining paper and electronic documents, etc., and analyze the results. (Evaluate)

3. *Communication techniques*
   Define and apply appropriate interviewing techniques (e.g., when to use various question types, the significance of pauses and their length, when and how to prompt a response), in various situations, such as when supervisors are present, when conducting multiple interviews, and when using a translator. Identify typical conflict situations and appropriate techniques for resolving them. (Apply)

4. *Working papers*
   Identify types of working papers, such as completed checklists, auditor notes, and attendance rosters, and determine their importance in providing evidence for an audit trail. (Create)

5. *Objective evidence*
   Identify and differentiate various characteristics of objective evidence, such as observed, measured, verified, and documented. (Evaluate)

6. *Observations*
   Evaluate the significance of observations in terms of positive, negative, chronic, isolated, and systemic. (Evaluate) [NOTE: This topic area includes general audit observation classification only; FDA classification criteria are covered in Body of Knowledge area II.E.3.]

7. *Classifying nonconformances*
   Classify nonconformances in terms of significance, severity, frequency, and level of risk. (Analyze)

8. *Audit process management*
   Define and apply elements of managing an audit, including coordinating team activities, reallocating resources, adjusting the audit plan, and communicating with the auditee during the audit. (Apply)

9. *Exit meeting*
   Describe the purpose and scope of an exit meeting and the necessary elements for conducting such a meeting, including determining post-audit activities and who is responsible for performing them. (Apply)

C. *Audit reporting*

1. *Basic elements*
   Define, plan, and apply the steps in generating an audit report, including reviewing and finalizing results, organizing details, obtaining necessary approvals, and distributing the report. (Create)

2. *Effective audit reports*
   Report observations and nonconformances accurately, cite objective evidence, procedures, and requirements, and develop and evaluate various components, such as executive summaries, prioritized data, graphic presentation, and the impact of conclusions. (Create)

3. *Record retention*
   Identify and apply record retention requirements, including the type of documents and storage considerations, for various audits. (Apply)

D. *Audit follow-up and closure*

1. *Elements of corrective and preventive action*
   Identify and apply the elements of these processes, including problem identification, assignment of responsibility, root cause analysis, and recurrence prevention. (Analyze)

2. *Review of corrective action plan*
   Use various criteria to evaluate the acceptability of corrective action plans, and identify and apply strategies for negotiating changes to unacceptable plans. (Evaluate)

3. *Conducting audit follow-up.*
   Use various methods to verify and evaluate the adequacy of corrective actions taken, such as re-examining procedures, observing revised processes, and conducting follow-up audits or re-audits. Develop strategies when corrective actions are not implemented or are not effective, such as communicating to the next level of management, re-issuing the corrective action request, etc. (Evaluate)

4. *Audit closure*
   Identify and apply various elements of, and criteria for, audit closure. (Evaluate)

E. *Audit procedural references*
1. *Guidelines for auditing quality systems*
    Describe general auditing principles and approaches as described in the ISO 19011 standard. (Understand)
2. *Quality System Inspection Technique (QSIT)*
    Explain the purpose of QSIT and its related terms, and compare QSIT to other audit approaches. Differentiate the principal subsystems of QSIT, and use and interpret QSIT sampling tables. (Analyze)
3. *US compliance programs for medical devices (FDA CPG 7382.845)*
    Explain the purpose and scope of various FDA inspections, including the criteria for the FDA taking action as a result of quality system audits, and categorize observations according to FDA classification criteria. (Apply)
    [NOTE: This topic area includes FDA classification criteria only; general audit observation classification is covered in Body of Knowledge area II.B.6.]
4. *International auditing guidelines for medical devices (GHTF SG4 (99)28, GHTF SG4 (99)14, GHTF SG4 (00)3)*
    Apply general auditing principles for medical device audits. Assess the adequacy of auditors' training, their qualifications to conduct audits of a medical device manufacturer's quality system, and ongoing training to maintain their qualifications. Assess an audit team's ability to read, speak, write, and understand the native language used by auditee personnel and the auditee's quality system documentation; assess the team's ability to arrange for an interpreter in advance of the audit. (Apply)

III. Biomedical Quality Management System Requirements [50 Questions]

A. *Regulatory requirements & guidance*
1. *European directive: Medical Device Directive 93/42/EEC of 14 June 1993 (Article 1)*
    Interpret the applications of the directive. (Understand)
2. *US requirements (FD&C Act, sections 301–304, 501–502, 704, 518, 513)*
    Identify how the FD&C Act defines and is applied to medical devices and differentiate between device classifications and pre-market requirements. Define misbranding and adulteration and the implications of each. Describe the FDA's authority to perform establishment inspections and mandate product recalls. (Apply)
3. *Labeling: 21 CFR 801, subpart A*
    Apply general labeling provisions for medical devices. (Apply)
4. *Establishment registration and device listing: 21 CFR 807*
    Define these requirements. (Understand)
5. *Electronic records and electronic signatures: 21 CFR 11*
    Define these requirements. (Understand)
6. *FDA guideline for the manufacture of in vitro diagnostic (IVD) products (Jan 10, 1994)*

Define IVD devices and other terms related to the use of good manufacturing practices (GMPs) for IVDs. (Understand)

B. *Quality systems regulations & standards*
1. *21 CFR 820*
Identify FDA explanations and justifications for the content of the QSReg from the preamble; apply the scope and defined terms to medical devices. (Understand)
2. *ISO 9001, ISO 9002, ISO 13485, ISO 13488*
Evaluate the selection, interpretation, and implementation of these various quality system standards. (Evaluate)
3. *GHTF.SG3.N99-8*
Evaluate the selection and use of this guidance for an auditee's quality system. (Evaluate)

C. *Management controls*
Examine management responsibility for the quality system, including organization, resources, management review, quality audits, and personnel requirements. (Analyze)

D. *Design controls*
Evaluate the scope and purpose of design control elements and implementation of a design control system. Assess the design control system for compliance to the Medical Device Directive (MDD), including Essential Requirements, harmonized standards, risk analysis, and clinical investigation. (Evaluate)

E. *Corrective and preventive actions (CAPA)*
1. *Existing and potential problem resolution*
Distinguish correction, corrective action, and preventive action, and explain their importance in terms of management responsibility, methods of implementing these tools, etc. Describe how trending is used as it relates to corrective and preventive action data. (Evaluate)
2. *Identification and control of nonconforming product (820.90)*
Define and apply various methods for detecting and controlling nonconforming product. (Analyze)
3. *Post-market surveillance*
Review and analyze complaint handling and servicing processes. Distinguish between vigilance and medical device reporting (MDR) requirements and processes. Evaluate the requirements and processes for product recall, corrections, removals, and medical device tracking. (Evaluate)

F. *Production and process controls (P&PC)*
1. *Document and change control (820.40, 820.180–820.186)*
Identify and distinguish between device master records (DMRs), design history files (DHFs), device history records (DHRs), and quality system records. Explain document and change control. (Analyze)
2. *Purchasing controls and acceptance activities (820.50, 820.80, [including product identification & traceability] 820.60, 820.65)*

Explain the importance of having adequate controls in purchasing products, components, and services, and the use of appropriate identification and acceptance activities. (Understand)

3. *Handling, storage, distribution and installation (820.140–820.170)*
Identify the requirements for these processes. (Understand)

4. *Validation and process controls (820.70, 820.75, 820.72, GHTF.SG3.N99-10)*
Assess a validation process and production and process controls in relation to components, materials, technology, product use, industry standards, production standards, test methods, and calibration. (Evaluate)

5. *Packaging and labeling controls (820.120, 820.130)*
Identify these requirements. (Understand)

6. *Sampling techniques (820.250(b))*
Identify, interpret, and use various sampling methods, such as acceptance, random, and stratified, and define related concepts (e.g., consumer and producer risk, and confidence level), as used in the biomedical field. (Apply)

7. *Statistical techniques (820.250(a))*
Identify, interpret, and use various measures of central tendency (mean, median, and mode), and dispersion, such as standard deviation and frequency distribution. Identify appropriate rationales for statistical techniques used in the biomedical field. (Apply)

IV. Technical Biomedical Knowledge [25 Questions]

A. *Risk management*
Identify the steps necessary for risk analysis of medical devices. Identify known or foreseeable hazards for medical devices in both normal and fault conditions, and describe suitable methods for risk estimation. Evaluate risk analysis reports for completeness, and use FMEA, FTA, and other tools to assess risk in a variety of situations. (Evaluate)

B. *Sterilization*

1. *Definitions*
Distinguish between aseptically processed products and terminally sterilized products. (Understand)

2. *Standards*
Identify the standards applicable to each sterilization process, including ISO 11134, ISO 11135, ISO 11137, ISO 11737, ISO 11138, ISO/TIR 13409, EN 550/552/554, and EN 556. (Understand)

3. *Methods*
Identify elements of sterilization validation, including commissioning of equipment installation and process qualification (physical and microbiological) and determine appropriateness. Identify appropriate process controls and monitors for each sterilization process and determine whether they are incorporated and documented properly. (Understand)

4. *Packaging of sterile products*
Interpret the appropriate standard for sterile product packaging, including ISO 11607 and EN 868-1. (Understand)

C. *Biocompatibility*
Define various biocompatibility terms, associated tests, and test selection rationale in accordance with ISO 10993, FDA Blue Book #G95-1, and U.S. Pharmacopoeia (USP) Classes V & VI. (Understand)

D. *Controlled environments and utility systems*

1. *Controlled environments*
Apply appropriate controlled environment classes for various medical devices. Identify and interpret controlled environment specifications as required by ISO 14644 and Federal Standard 209 E. Interpret qualifications, validation, and monitoring, including cleaning, disinfection, and sanitization in terms of controlled environment specifications, classifications, and standards. Verify that appropriate training and personnel practices are in use for controlled environments. (Evaluate)

2. *Utility systems*
Recognize water, compressed gas, and HVAC utilities used in medical device manufacturing and determine whether they require qualification, validation, or maintenance according to U.S. Pharmacopoeia (USP), ISO 14644, Federal Standard 209E, or ISO 11134 standards. (Understand)

E. *Software development for products, processes, and quality systems*
Define the major elements of software development, such as requirements specifications, unit testing, integration and systems testing, verification, validation, etc., in accordance with FDA software Guidance for FDA Reviewers and Industry, (May 29, 1998), General Principles of Software Validation, 21 CFR Part 11, and ISPE Good Automated Manufacturing Practice (GAMP4) requirements. (Understand)

F. *Laboratory testing*
Review validation procedures used for laboratory test methods and determine whether they are appropriate. (Evaluate)

V. Quality Tools & Techniques [15 Questions]

A. *Fundamental quality control tools*
Interpret and apply Pareto charts, cause and effect diagrams, flowcharts, control charts, check sheets, scatter diagrams, and histograms. (Apply)

B. *Quality improvement tools*
Interpret and apply problem-solving tools, such as root cause analysis, the six sigma model (DMAIC), lean tools, Plan–Do–Check–Act (PDCA), and corrective and preventive action (CAPA) methods. (Apply)

C. *Process capability*
Identify and interpret various process capability indices, such as Cp and Cpk. (Understand)

    D. *Qualitative and quantitative analysis*
        Describe and distinguish between qualitative and quantitative analyses, and attributes and variables data. (Analyze)

    E. *Cost of quality*
        Identify the basic cost of quality (COQ) principles, and describe the four COQ categories. (Understand)

LEVELS OF COGNITION BASED ON BLOOM'S TAXONOMY—REVISED (2001)

In addition to *content* specifics, the subtext for each topic in this Body of Knowledge also indicates the intended *complexity level* of the test questions for that topic. These levels are based on "Levels of Cognition" (from Bloom's Taxonomy—Revised, 2001) and are presented below in rank order, from least complex to most complex.

Remember (Knowledge Level)

Recall or recognize terms, definitions, facts, ideas, materials, patterns, sequences, methods, principles, etc.

Understand (Comprehension Level)

Read and understand descriptions, communications, reports, tables, diagrams, directions, regulations, etc.

Apply (Application Level)

Know when and how to use ideas, procedures, methods, formulas, principles, theories, etc.

Analyze (Analysis Level)

Break down information into its constituent parts and recognize their relationship to one another and how they are organized; identify sublevel factors or salient data from a complex scenario.

Evaluate (Evaluation Level)

Make judgments about the value of proposed ideas, solutions, etc., by comparing the proposal to specific criteria or standards.

Create (Synthesis Level)

Put parts or elements together in such a way as to reveal a pattern or structure not clearly there before; identify which data or information from a complex set is appropriate to examine further or from which supported conclusions can be drawn.

Appendix B
Glossary of Terms

absorbed dose—the quantity of radiation energy imparted per unit mass of matter. The unit of absorbed dose is the gray (Gy) where one gray is equivalent to absorption of one joule per kilogram.

accessory—an article that, while not being a device, is intended specifically by its manufacturer to be used together with a device to enable it to be used in accordance with the use of the device intended by the manufacturer of the device.

act—the FDCA, 21 USC 321 et seq., as amended.

active implantable medical device—any active medical device that is intended to be totally or partially introduced, surgically or medically, into the human body or by medical intervention into a natural orifice, and that is intended to remain after the procedure.

active medical device—any medical device relying for its functioning on a source of electrical energy or any source of power other than that directly generated by the human body or gravity.

aeration—the removal of ethylene oxide and its reaction products (such as ethylene chlorhydrin) from a medical device using forced warm air ventilation.

aseptic—a process in which sterile product is packaged in sterile containers in a manner that avoids contamination of the product, for example, the aseptic filling of sterile vials with sterile liquid.

audit—a systematic and independent examination to determine whether quality activities and related results comply with planned arrangements and whether these arrangements are implemented effectively and are suitable to achieve objectives.

audit language—the language(s) routinely used for the communication or exchange of information between auditee's personnel and auditors.

auditee—any organization whose quality systems are to be audited for compliance with the relevant medical device regulatory requirements.

auditing organization—a body designated, on the basis of specific regulations, to carry out audits according to assigned tasks.

auditor—a person with relevant qualifications and competence to perform audits or specified parts of such audits and who belongs to, or is authorized by, the auditing organization.

authorized representative—any natural or legal person established in the community who, explicitly designated by the manufacturer, acts and may be addressed by authorities and bodies in the community instead of the manufacturer with regard to the latter's obligations under this directive.

bacteriostasis/fungistasis test—a test that utilizes selected microorganisms to demonstrate the presence of substances that may inhibit the multiplication of the microorganisms.

batch—a defined quantity of bulk, intermediate, or finished product that is intended or purported to be uniform in character and quality, and which has been produced during a defined cycle of manufacture.

bioburden—the population of living microorganisms, bacterial and fungal, on a raw material, component, finished product, or package.

biological indicator—a carrier inoculated with a known microorganism with a known resistance to the sterilization process under study.

calibration—the comparison of a measurement system or device of unknown accuracy to a measurement system or device of known accuracy to detect, correlate, report, or eliminate by adjustment any variation from the required performance limits of the unverified measurement system or device.

commissioning—developing the evidence that equipment has been provided and installed in accordance with its specification and that it functions within predetermined limits when operated in accordance with operational instructions.

complaint—any written, electronic, or oral communication that alleges deficiencies related to the identity, quality, durability, reliability, safety, effectiveness, or performance of a device after it is released for distribution.

component—any raw material, substance, piece, part, software, firmware, labeling, or assembly that is intended to be included as part of the finished, packaged, and labeled device.

contract sterilizer—any facility that offers to provide a contractual service intended to sterilize products that are manufactured by another establishment.

control number—any distinctive symbols, such as a distinctive combination of letters or numbers, or both, from which the history of the manufacturing, packaging, labeling, and distribution of a unit, lot, or batch of finished devices can be determined.

correction—an action taken to eliminate a detected nonconformity (for example, repair or rework). A correction can be taken in conjunction with a corrective action.

corrective action—an action taken to eliminate the cause of a detected nonconformity or other undesirable situation. Corrective action is taken to prevent recurrence of a nonconformity.

D value—the exposure time to a sterilizing process that is required to produce a 1-logarithm or 90 percent reduction in the population of a microorganism, usually an indicator organism.

design history file (DHF)—a compilation of records that describes the design history of a finished device.

design input—the physical and performance requirements of a device that are used as a basis for device design.

design output—the results of a design effort at each design phase and at the end of the total design effort. The finished design output is the basis for the device master record. The total finished design output consists of the device, its packaging and labeling, and the device master record.

design review—a documented, comprehensive, systematic examination of a design to evaluate the adequacy of the design requirements, to evaluate the capability of the design to meet these requirements, and to identify problems.

design validation—establishing by objective evidence that device specifications conform with user needs and intended use(s).

device failure—the failure of a device to perform or function as intended, including any deviations from the device's performance specifications or intended use.

device for self-testing—any device intended by the manufacturer to be able to be used by lay persons in a home environment.

device history record (DHR)—a compilation of records containing the production history of a finished device.

device master record (DMR)—a compilation of records containing the procedures and specifications for a finished device.

directions for use—This term provides directions under which the practitioner or layman (for example, patient or unlicensed health care provider), as appropriate, can use the device safely and for the purposes for which it is intended. Directions for use also include indications for use and appropriate contraindications, warnings, precautions, and adverse reaction information. Directions for use requirements applicable to prescription and over-the-counter devices appear throughout 21 CFR Part 801 and, in the case of in vitro diagnostic products, under 21 CFR 809.10.

distributes—any distribution of a tracked device, including the charitable distribution of a tracked device. This term does not include the distribution of a device under an effective investigational device exemption in accordance with section 520(g) of the act and part 812 of this chapter or the distribution of a device for teaching, law enforcement, research, or analysis as specified in Section 801.125 of this chapter.

distributor—any person who furthers the distribution of a device from the original place of manufacture to the person who makes delivery or sale to the ultimate user, that is, the final or multiple distributor, but who does not repackage or otherwise change the container, wrapper, or labeling of the device or device package.

dosimeter—a device or system having a reproducible measurable response to radiation, which can be used to measure the absorbed dose in a given material.

environmental controls—those controls and standardized procedures used in the manufacturing areas to control bioburden levels. Such controls may include air filters, fluid filters, use of surface disinfectants, personnel gowning or uniforms, and personnel training.

establish—define, document (in writing or electronically), and implement.

F value—a measure of the effectiveness of a heat sterilization process to inactivate living microorganisms. The F value is calculated by determining the lethal rate per minute at each process temperature using the z value of the microorganisms.

F_0 value—the F value of a heat sterilization process calculated at 121.1° C with a z value of 10 K and a D value of one minute.

final distributor—any person who distributes a tracked device intended for use by a single patient over the useful life of the device to the patient. This term includes, but is not limited to, licensed practitioners, retail pharmacies, hospitals, and other types of device user facilities.

finished device—any device or accessory to any device that is suitable for use or capable of functioning, whether or not it is packaged, labeled, or sterilized.

importer—the initial distributor of an imported device who is required to register under section 510 of the act and Section 807.20 of this chapter. "Importer" does not include anyone who only performs a service for the person who furthers the marketing, that is, brokers, jobbers, or warehousers.

in vitro diagnostic medical device—any medical device that is a reagent, reagent product, calibrator, control material, kit, instrument, apparatus, equipment, or system, whether used alone or in combination, intended by the manufacturer to be used in vitro for the examination of specimens, including blood and tissue donations, derived from the human body, solely or principally for the purpose of providing information: 1) concerning a physiological or pathological state; 2) concerning a congenital abnormality; 3) to determine the safety and compatibility with potential recipients; or 4) to monitor therapeutic measures.

Specimen receptacles are considered to be in vitro diagnostic medical devices. Specimen receptacles are those devices, whether vacuum-type or not, specifically intended by their manufacturers for the primary containment and preservation of specimens derived from the human body for the purpose of in vitro diagnostic examination.

Products for general laboratory use are not in vitro diagnostic medical devices unless such products, in view of their characteristics, are specifically intended by their manufacturer to be used for in vitro diagnostic examination.

installation qualification—a step in the sterilization validation program that establishes, using appropriate studies and records, that the process equipment can perform within its design specifications.

intended uses—The term "intended uses" refers to the objective intent of the persons legally responsible for the labeling of the device. The intent is determined by their expressions or may be shown by the circumstances surrounding the distribution of the device. This objective intent may, for example, be shown by labeling claims, advertising matter, or oral or written statements by such representatives. It may be shown by the offering or the using of the device, with the knowledge of such persons or their representatives, for a purpose for which it is neither labeled nor advertised. (21 CFR 801.4)

IVD accessory—an article that, while not being an in vitro diagnostic medical device, is intended specifically by its manufacturer to be used together with a device to enable that device to be used in accordance with its intended purpose.

Invasive sampling devices or those that are directly applied to the human body for the purpose of obtaining a specimen within the meaning of Directive 93/42/EEC shall not be considered to be accessories to in vitro diagnostic medical devices.

label—a display of written, printed, or graphic matter upon the immediate container of any article. [section 201(k).]

labeling—includes all labels and other written, printed, or graphic matter: 1) upon any article or any of its containers or wrappers; or 2) accompanying such article. [section 201(m).]

lead auditor—an auditor designated to manage an audit (also known as an audit team leader).

licensed practitioner—a physician, dentist, or other healthcare practitioner licensed by the law of the state in which he or she practices to use or order the use of the tracked device. (m) Any term defined in section 201 of the act shall have the same definition in this part.

life-supporting or life-sustaining device (used outside a device user facility)—a device that is essential, or yields information that is essential, to the restoration or continuation of a bodily function important to the continuation of human life that is intended for use outside a hospital, nursing home, ambulatory surgical facility, or diagnostic or outpatient treatment facility. Physicians' offices are not device user facilities and, therefore, devices used therein are subject to tracking if they otherwise satisfy the statutory and regulatory criteria.

lot or batch—one or more components or finished devices that consist of a single type, model, class, size, composition, or software version that are manufactured under essentially the same conditions and are intended to have uniform characteristics and quality within specified limits.

management with executive responsibility—senior employees of a manufacturer who have the authority to establish or make changes to the manufacturer's quality policy and quality system.

manufacturer—any person who designs, manufactures, fabricates, assembles, or processes a finished device. Manufacturer includes, but is not limited to, those who perform the functions of contract sterilization, installation, relabeling, remanufacturing, repacking, or specification development, and initial distributors of foreign entities performing these functions.

manufacturer (ISO)—the natural or legal person with responsibility for the design, manufacture, packaging, and labeling of a device before it is placed on the market under his own name, regardless of whether these operations are carried out by that person or on his or her behalf by a third party. The obligations of this directive to be met by manufacturers also apply to the natural or legal person who assembles, packages, processes, fully refurbishes, and/or labels one or more ready-made products and/or assigns to them their intended purpose as devices with a view to their being placed on the market under his or her own name. This subparagraph does not apply to the person who, while not a manufacturer within the meaning of the first subparagraph, assembles or adapts devices already on the market to their intended purpose for an individual patient.

manufacturing material—any material or substance used in or used to facilitate the manufacturing process, a concomitant constituent, or a byproduct constituent produced during the manufacturing process, which is present in or on the finished device as a residue or impurity not by design or intent of the manufacturer.

medical device—any instrument, apparatus, appliance, material, or other article, whether used alone or in combination, including the software necessary for its proper application, intended by the manufacturer to be used for human beings for the purpose of:

- Diagnosis, prevention, monitoring, treatment, or alleviation of disease

- Diagnosis, monitoring, treatment, alleviation, or compensation for an injury or handicap

- Investigation, replacement or modification of the anatomy or of a physiological process

- Control of conception

and that does not achieve its principal intended action in or on the human body by pharmacological, immunological, or metabolic means, but which may be assisted in its function by such means.

microbiological challenge—a population of known microorganisms, such as biological indicators, biological indicator test packs, or inoculated product, that can be used to test a sterilization cycle.

multiple distributor—any device user facility, rental company, or any other entity that distributes a life-sustaining or life-supporting device intended for use by more than one patient over the useful life of the device.

nonconformity—the nonfulfillment of a specified requirement.

objective evidence—verifiable information or records pertaining to the quality of an item or service or to the existence and implementation of a quality system element, which is based on visual observation, measurement, or test.

parametric release—a method of declaring that a product is sterile based on a review of the process data rather than on the basis of sample testing or biological indicator results.

permanently implantable device—a device that is intended to be placed into a surgically or naturally formed cavity of the human body to continuously assist, restore, or replace the function of an organ system or structure of the human body throughout the useful life of the device. The term does not include any device that is intended and used for temporary purposes or that is intended for explanation.

preconditioning—a step in the sterilization process prior to exposure to the sterilizing gas mixture, designed to bring the product to specified conditions of temperature and relative humidity. This step may be accomplished within the sterilization vessel, in an external area, or in both.

presterilization count—population of viable microorganisms on a product or package prior to sterilization.

preventive action—an action taken to eliminate the cause of a potential nonconformity or other undesirable potential situation. Preventive action is taken to prevent occurrence of a nonconformity.

process qualification—obtaining and documenting evidence that the sterilization process will produce acceptable products.

process validation—establishing by objective evidence that a process consistently produces a result or product meeting its predetermined specifications.

product—components, manufacturing materials, in-process devices, finished devices, and returned devices.

pyrogen—a biological or chemical agent that produces a fever in mammals.

quality—the totality of features and characteristics that bear on the ability of a device to satisfy fitness for use, including safety and performance.

quality audit—a systematic, independent examination of a manufacturer's quality system that is performed at defined intervals and at sufficient frequency to determine whether both quality system activities and the results of such activities comply with quality system procedures, that these procedures are implemented effectively, and that these procedures are suitable to achieve quality system objectives.

quality audit observation—statement of fact made during a quality audit and substantiated by objective evidence.

quality policy—the overall intentions and direction of an organization with respect to quality, as established by management with executive responsibility.

quality system—the organizational structure, responsibilities, procedures, processes, and resources for implementing quality management.

quality system record—procedures and the documentation of activities required by this part that are not specific to a particular device(s), including but not limited to the records required by § 820.20.

recovery efficiency—measure of the ability of a specific technique to remove and culture microorganisms from a test article.

regulatory requirements—any part of a law, ordinance, decree, or other regulation that applies to quality systems of medical device manufacturers. Guidelines, notes, draft documents, or the like should not be used as regulatory documents and are not to be construed as such unless formally promulgated.

remanufacturer—any person who processes, conditions, renovates, repackages, restores, or does any other act to a finished device that significantly changes the finished device's performance or safety specifications, or intended use.

rework—action taken on a nonconforming product so that it will fulfill the specified DMR requirements before it is released for distribution.

serious adverse health consequences—any significant adverse experience related to a device, including device-related events that are life-threatening or that involve permanent or long-term injuries or illnesses.

simulated product load—A sterilization vessel load that is as difficult to sterilize as the actual product load.

specification—any requirement with which a product, process, service, or other activity must conform.

sterile—free from living microorganisms. In practice, sterility is expressed as a probability function. For example, sterility may be expressed as the probability of a surviving microorganism as being one in a million (10^{-6}).

sterility assurance level (SAL)—the probability of a nonsterile product after sterilization. The SAL is usually expressed as 10^{-n}.

sterilization—the process used to remove all living microorganisms on a product.

sterilization dose—the minimum absorbed dose of radiation required to achieve the specified sterility assurance level.

temperature distribution study—a study to determine the temperature profile within a sterilizing chamber during a sterilization cycle.

terminal sterilization—the process in which the product is rendered free of microorganisms at the last stage(s) of the manufacturing process. In the case of ethylene oxide and radiation sterilization, the product is typically sterilized in the final packaging, including the shipping containers. In the case of moist heat sterilization, the product is sterilized in the primary container with subsequent label application and final packaging.

training elements—topics within a training program that describe the content for addressing a particular training need.

21 CFR § 807.3 (b) **commercial distribution**—any distribution of a device intended for human use that is held or offered for sale but does not include the following: 1) internal or interplant transfer of a device between establishments within the same parent, subsidiary, and/or affiliate company; 2) any distribution of a device intended for human use that has in effect an approved exemption for investigational use under section 520(g) of the act and part 812 of this chapter; 3) any distribution of a device, before the effective date of part 812 of this chapter, that was not introduced or delivered for introduction into interstate commerce for commercial distribution before May 28, 1976, and that is classified into class III under section 513(f) of the act, provided, that the device is intended solely for investigational use, and under section 501(f)(2)(A) of the act the device is not required to have an approved premarket approval application as provided in section 515 of the act; or 4) for foreign establishments, the distribution of any device that is neither imported nor offered for import into the United States.

21 CFR § 807.3 (c) **establishment**—a place of business under one management at one general physical location at which a device is manufactured, assembled, or otherwise processed.

21 CFR § 807.3 (e) **official correspondent**—the person designated by the owner or operator of an establishment as responsible for the following: 1) the annual registration of the establishment; 2) contact with the FDA for device listing; 3) maintenance and submission of a current list of officers and directors to the FDA upon the request of the commissioner; 4) the receipt of pertinent correspondence from the FDA directed to and involving the owner or operator and/or any of the firm's establishments; and 5) the annual certification of MDRs required by Section 804.30 of this chapter or forwarding the certification form to the person designated by the firm as responsible for the certification.

21 CFR § 807.3 (f) **owner or operator**—the corporation, subsidiary, affiliated company, partnership, or proprietor directly responsible for the activities of the registering establishment.

21 CFR § 807.3 (g) **initial importer**—any importer who furthers the marketing of a device from a foreign manufacturer to the person who makes the final delivery or sale of the device to the ultimate consumer or user, but does not repackage, or otherwise change the container, wrapper, or labeling of the device or device package.

21 CFR § 807.3 (r) **United States agent**—a person residing in or maintaining a place of business in the United States whom a foreign establishment designates as its agent. This definition excludes mailboxes, answering machines, or services, or other places where an individual acting as the foreign establishment's agent is not physically present.

validation—confirmation by examination and provision of objective evidence that the particular requirements for a specific intended use can be consistently fulfilled.

verification—confirmation by examination and provision of objective evidence that specified requirements have been fulfilled.

where appropriate—when a requirement is qualified by "where appropriate," it is deemed to be appropriate unless the manufacturer can document justification otherwise.

z value—the number of degrees of temperature required for a 1-logarithm change in the D value. A z value can be obtained from a thermal resistance curve; D values are plotted against temperature, and the reciprocal of the slope is determined as the z value.

References

American Standard, ASQ D1160, Formal Design Review.

Electronic records; electronic signatures, 21 CFR, pt.11 (2002).

Enforcement policy, 21 CFR, pt. 7 (2002).

Establishment registration and device listing for manufacturers and initial importers of devices, 21 CFR, pt. 807 (2002).

European Standard, 93/42/EEC, Medical Devices.

European Standard, BS EN 552, Sterilization of Medical Devices—Validation and Routine Control of Sterilization by Irradiation.

European Standard, BS EN 554, Sterilization of Medical Devices—Validation and Routine Control of Sterilization by Moist Heat.

European Standard, DIN EN 550, Sterilization of Medical Devices; Validation and Routine Control of Ethylene Oxide Sterilization.

European Standard, EN 46001, Quality Systems—Medical Devices—Particular Requirements for the Application of EN 29001.

European Standard, EN 556, Sterilization of Medical Devices—Requirements for Terminally-Sterilized Devices to Be Labelled "Sterile."

European Standard, EN 868-1, Packaging Materials for Sterilization of Wrapped Goods—Part 1: General Requirements and Requirements for the Validation of Packaging for Terminally Sterilized Devices.

FDA. Compliance Policy Guide section 160.850, Enforcement Policy: 21 CFR Part 11; Electronic records; Electronic Signatures. (Food and Drug Administration [FDA], Office of Regulatory Affairs, 13 May 1999).

FDA. General Principles of Software Validation; Final Guidance for Industry and FDA Staff. (Food and Drug Administration [FDA], Center for Devices and Radiological Health, January 11, 2002).

FDA. General Principles of Software Validation; Final Guidance for Industry and FDA Staff. (Food and Drug Administration [FDA], Center for Devices and Radiological Health, January 11, 2002).

FDA. Guidance for FDA Reviewers and Industry Guidance for the Content of Premarket Submissions for Software Contained in Medical Devices. (Food and Drug Administration [FDA], Center for Devices and Radiological Health, May 29, 1998).

FDA. Guide to Inspections of Quality Systems. (Food and Drug Administration [FDA], Center for Devices and Radiological Health, August 1999).

FDA. Guideline for the Manufacture of In Vitro Diagnostic Products. (Food and Drug Administration [FDA], Center for Devices and Radiological Health, January 10, 1994).

FDA. Inspection of Medical Device Manufacturers, Final Guidance for Industry and FDA. (Food and Drug Administration [FDA], Center for Devices and Radiological Health, February 7, 2001).

FDA. Required Biocompatibility Training and Toxicology Profiles for Evaluation of Medical Devices. (Food and Drug Administration [FDA], Office of Regulatory Affairs, May 1, 1995 [G95-1]).

Food and Drugs, 21 US Code.

General Labeling Provisions, 21 CFR, pt. 801 subpt. A (2002)

Global Harmonization Task Force. SG2-N21R8: Adverse Event Reporting Guidance for the Medical Device Manufacturer or Its Authorized Representative.

Global Harmonization Task Force. SG3-N99-10: Process Validation Guidance for Medical Device Manufacturers.

Global Harmonization Task Force. SG4 (00) 3: Training Requirements for Auditors.

Global Harmonization Task Force. SG4 (99) 14: Audit Language Requirements.

Global Harmonization Task Force. SG4 (99) 28: Guidelines for Regulatory Auditing of Quality Systems of Medical Device Manufacturers—Part 1: General Requirements.

Internation Standard, ANSI/ISO/ASQ Q9001-2000, Quality Management Systems: Requirements.

International Standard ANSI/AAMI/ISO 10993-1, Biological evaluation of medical devices—Part 1; Evaluation and Testing.

International Standard ISO 14644-1, Cleanrooms and Associated Controlled Environments—Part 1. Classification of Air Cleanliness.

International Standard, ANSI/ISO/IEC 17025, General Requirements for the Competence of Testing and Calibration Laboratories.

International Standard, IEC 60601-1-1, Medical Electrical Equipment—Part 1: General Requirements for Safety 1: Collateral Standard: Safety Requirements for Medical Electrical Systems.

International Standard, IEC 60601-1-4, Medical Electrical Equipment—Part 1–4. General Requirements for Safety—Collateral Standard: Programmable Electrical Medical Systems.

International Standard, ISO 11135, Medical devices—Validation and routine control of ethylene oxide sterilization.

International Standard, ISO 11137, Sterilization of health care products—Requirements for validation and routine control—Radiation sterilization.

International Standard, ISO 11138-1, Sterilization of health care products—Biological indicators—Part 1: General.

International Standard, ISO 11138-2, Sterilization of health care products—Biological indicators—Part 2: Biological indicators for ethylene oxide sterilization.

International Standard, ISO 11607, Packaging for terminally sterilized medical devices.

International Standard, ISO 13485:2003, Medical devices—Quality management systems—Requirements for regulatory purposes.

International Standard, ISO 14971, Medical Devices—Application of risk management to medical devices.

International Standard, ISO TR 13409, Sterilization of health care Products—Radiation sterilization—Substaniation of 25 Kgy as a sterilization dose for small or infrequent production batches.

Medical device reporting, 21 CFR, pt. 803 (2002)

Medical device tracking requirements, 21 CFR, pt. 821 (2002)

Medical devices; reports of corrections and removals, 21 CFR, pt. 806 (2002)

Military Standard (MIL STD)-882C. Military Standard System Safety Program Requirements (Department of Defense [DOD], 19 January 1993).

Quality system regulation, 21 CFR, pt. 810 (1997).

United States Pharmacopeial Convention, Inc. The United States Pharmacopeia/National Formulary.

WEB SITES

American Society for Quality http://www.asq.org
ASQ Biomedical Division http://www.asqbiomed.org
FDA Enforcement Report http://www.fda.gov/opacom/Enforce.html.
FDA Office Regulatory Assistance http://www.fda.gov.ora
FDA Safety Alerts http://www.fda.gov/cdrh/safety.html
Food and Drug Administration http://www.fda.gov
GMP References http://www.fda.gov/cdrh/dsma/cgmphome.html
Inspection Notice Form http://www.fda.gov/ora/inspect_ref/iom/exhibits/x510a.pdf
Inspection Operations Manual http://www.fda.gov/ora/inspect_ref/iom/default.htm
Inspection Operations Manual Index
    http://www.fda.gov/ora/inspect_ref/iom/iomoradir.html.
Other inspection resources http://www.fda.gov/ora/inspect_ref/default.htm

Index